JUN 0 5

D0567651

C   G

You   's

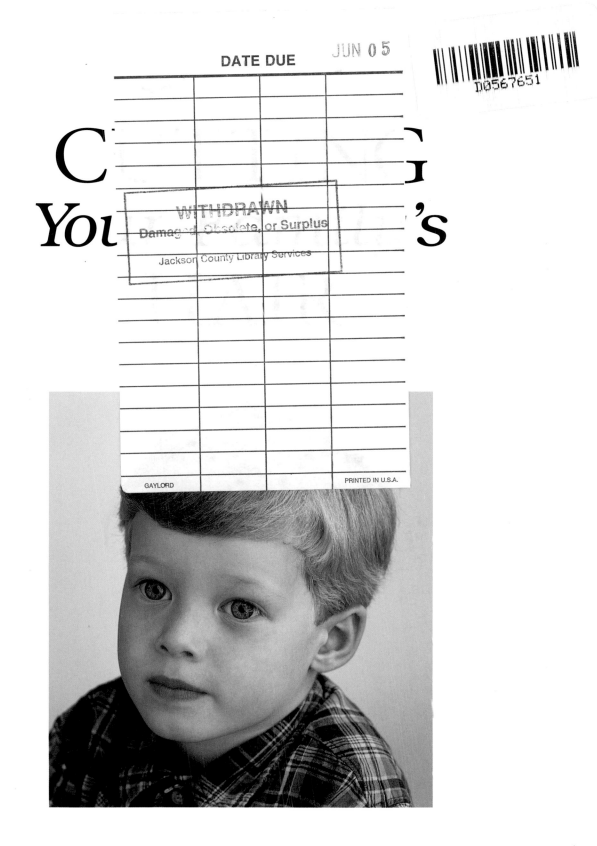

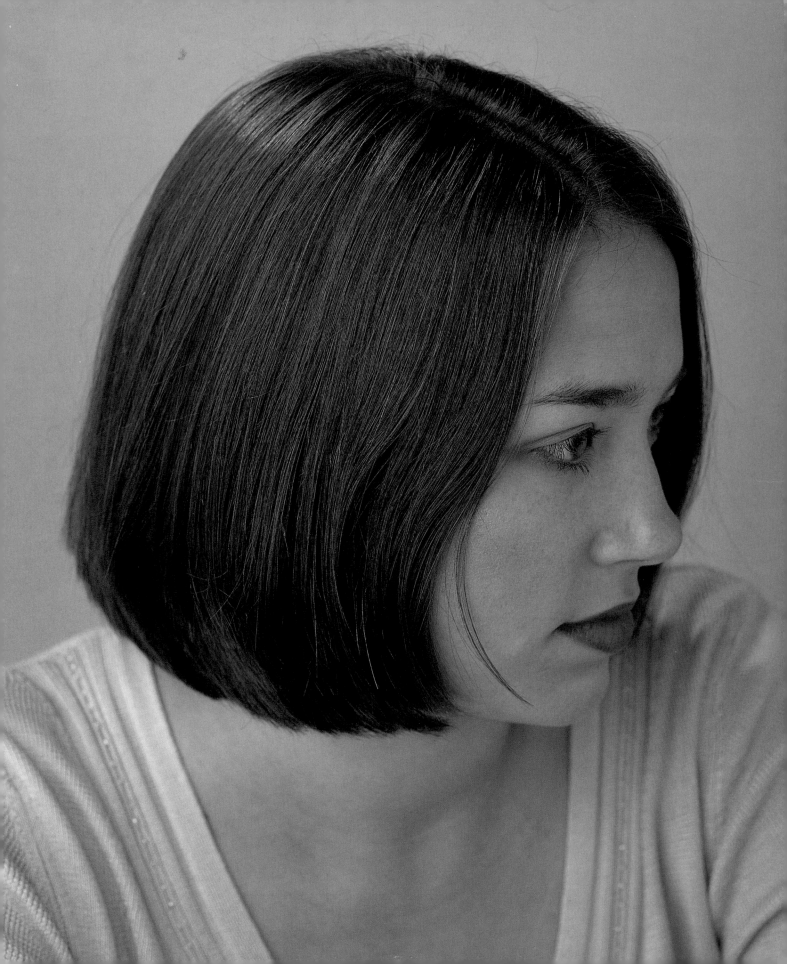

CUTTING
Your Family's
HAIR

Gloria Handel

Sterling Publishing Co., Inc.

Prolific Impressions Production Staff:

Editor in Chief: Mickey Baskett

Copy Editor: Phyllis Mueller

Graphics: Dianne Miller, Karen Turpin

Photography: Pat Molnar

Administration: Jim Baskett

Library of Congress Cataloging-in-Publication Data Available

10 9 8 7 6 5 4 3 2 1

Published by Sterling Publishing Company, Inc.
387 Park Avenue South, New York, N.Y. 10016

Produced by Prolific Impressions, Inc.
160 South Candler St., Decatur, GA 30030
©2002 by Prolific Impressions, Inc.
Distributed in Canada by Sterling Publishing
c/o Canadian Manda Group, One Atlantic Avenue, Suite 105
Toronto, Ontario, Canada M6K 3E7
Distributed in Great Britain and Europe by Cassell PLC
Wellington House, 125 Strand, London WC2R 0BB, England
Distributed in Australia by Capricorn Link (Australia) Pty. Ltd.
P.O. Box 704, Winsor, NSW 2756 Australia

Printed in China
All rights reserved
Sterling ISBN   0-8069-5851-0

ABOUT THE AUTHOR

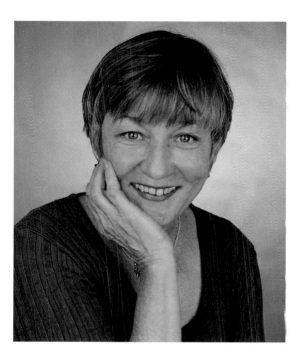

Gloria Handel is a freelance hairstylist, artist, and writer who lives and works in Decatur, Georgia, where she pursues her interests in hair care, art, and natural herbal products and herbal remedies. For ten years, she was the owner and proprietor of a hair salon and was named Decatur's Small Business Person of the Year in 1990.

Studying art – specifically painting and writing – has become a passion. Handel's artwork is an exploration in abstractions, using brush strokes and color to express feelings. Her paintings have been exhibited in numerous shows, including ones at The Atlanta College of Art and Emory University. She received a B.A. from Agnes Scott College in fine art in 1996.

Handel's love for the outdoors often takes her to Montana, where her daughter Shannon lives. She enjoys rafting, hiking, horseback riding, and photography. These adventures in the West inspire her paintings and writings. You may visit her website (http://home. earthlink.net/~ghandel3) to ask and receive answers to your questions concerning hair styling and hair care and to view her paintings.

Dedication

I want to dedicate this book to my mother and my grandmother, who encouraged me to pursue a career in cosmetology; to my sisters Sandra and Julene and my aunt Judy, who were my first clients; to my children and grandchildren, Matthew, Shannon, Courtnay, Drew, Ashlegh, Sarah, and Lindsay, for their loving support; and to all my clients over the years, who have been loyal to my service.

Acknowledgements

I would like to thank Mickey Baskett for making this book possible, Phyllis Mueller for editing, Deborah Ivester for doing the make-up, and all the models for their time and commitment to this project.

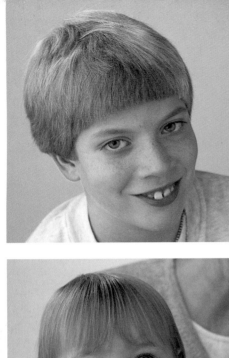

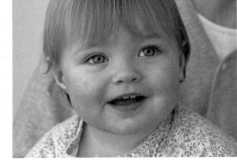

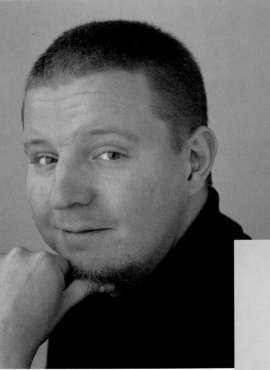

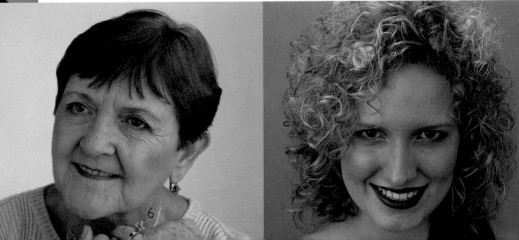

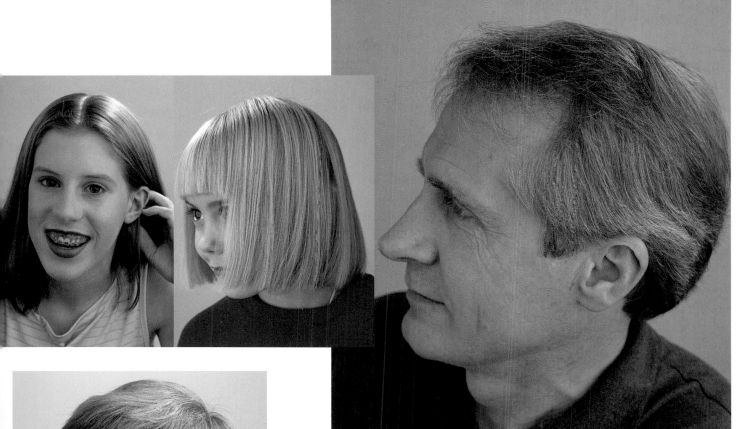

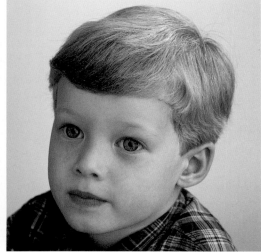

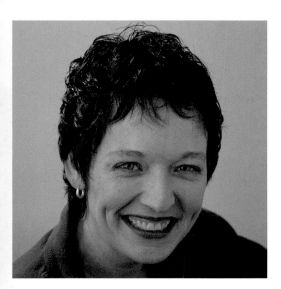

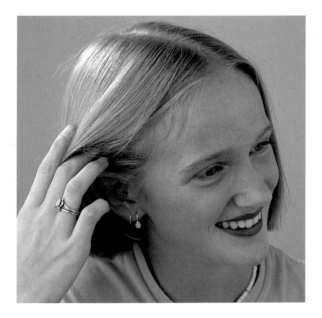

A Practical Guide to Haircutting and Hair Care for the Whole Family

Not only can you save time and money
by being able to cut the hair of your family members or friends;
but, you can give them the hair style they have been wanting.
Because you know them – their likes, dislikes, and personality
– you will be better equipped to find the hair style that
suits their lifestyle and their sense of self.
You can make them feel good and you will also be spending some
valuable time bonding with them. Nothing is more personal than
grooming, and you can have the opportunity for intimacy with your
family and friends by performing this special service for them.

This book will demystify the rules of haircutting for you.
We have presented some easy cuts that you can do in your home.
Once you learn the basic precepts, you will be able to cut any length
or style of hair your friend or family member desires. It's easy, fun, and
anyone can do it once you learn the techniques presented here.

History Plays a Big Part in Hair Grooming

There are several reasons why, in most societies, people cut and style their hair. Keeping it out of the way is the first and most practical reason we modify our hair from its natural state. Personal adornment is a basic desire most cultures observe, and hair is a key element. Through history hair has been a powerful symbol. Shamans and healers through time have used hair in ritual. In pre-industrial societies, hairstyles indicated social status; hairstyles in modern society often indicate social ordering.

The religious significance of hair is seen in the shaved heads of Christian and Buddhist monks, signifying their renunciation of the world. Muslim men anticipate that Allah will use their single lock of hair to pull them to heaven. The long curling locks of the Royalist Anglican Cavaliers and the cropped hair of the Parliamentarian Puritan Roundheads professed political and religious significance in 17th century England.

Historically, hair arrangement has proclaimed age and marital status. When boys in ancient Greece reached adolescence they cut their hair. Hindu boys shaved their heads. Matrons bound their hair under veils in medieval Europe, and young maidens wore uncovered, flowing hair. During mourning, heads in ancient Egypt that were usually shaven grew hair, and long-haired Hindu widows cut off their hair.

Since the middle ages hair styles in the West have been influenced by changing fashions. Courtiers in the 17th century wore wigs, following the lead of the balding Louis XIV. In the 20th century, women of all classes followed the example of film stars like Jean Harlow and wore platinum hair. Fashionable hair styles until the 20th century were generally reserved for the upper classes, and the dictates of fashion were relatively rigid. In modern society, due to increases in wealth, the trend toward individuality, and advances in mass communication, men and women generally choose the cut and style that best suits their needs and tastes.

Nobody Wants a Bad Hair Day

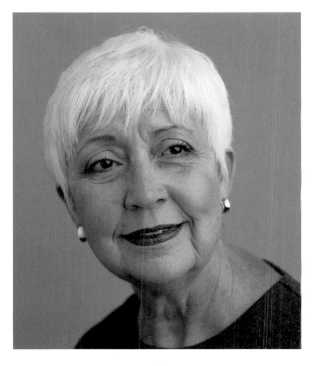

A perky cut can make us feel perky, while a sleek style feels sophisticated. On the other hand, a bad haircut has an adverse affect. To avoid having a bad hair day, it is important to understand how to develop skills for having healthy, well-cut hair. Basic haircutting skills are simple to learn. In the right environment and with the right tools, haircutting allows the cutter an opportunity to practice a skill and the ability to affect how others feel about themselves. There is always a creative edge to the haircutting process, but it is not necessary to feel creative in order to give a good haircut. Most importantly, it is a service of great value.

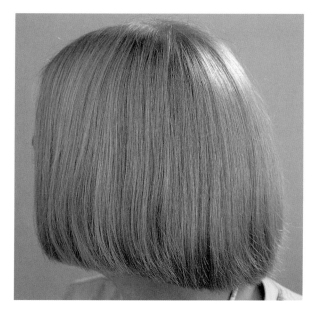

Healthy Hair Care

Beautiful, healthy, shiny hair can be yours if you accept the
kind of hair you have. Learning how to appreciate your
natural hair, whether thick or thin, curly or straight, is the first
step. Finding the right cut and hair care products is the
next crucial step.

Hair also needs to be kept clean because dirt, oil, sweat,
and products can build up on the hair and scalp. To
prevent loss or damage, avoid pulling the hair back in tight
braids or ponytails, brushing it harshly, or abusing it with
harsh chemicals.

How healthy the hair is always affects the final results of
the style. There are many foods, oils, herbs, and condiments
that can be used to cleanse, condition, and set the hair.
A healthy diet and vitamin and herbal supplements are
important for healthy hair and scalp.

FOODS & VITAMINS

Hair is made up of protein, oil, and moisture.
Keeping all three in balance is the secret to shiny,
healthy locks. Eating a well balanced diet, drinking lots
of water, and getting proper rest will be reflected in the
condition of the hair.

Nutritional deficiencies can be one cause of hair loss, along with stress, hormonal imbalances, heredity, protein deficiency, or liver problems. When we lack necessary nutrients, the hair will show signs of deficiencies – it may be as dramatic as hair loss or simply loss of luster.

With our busy lives and fast foods, it may be necessary to supplement our diets with vitamins, minerals, and herbs. For best results and a proper diagnosis, seek the advice of a qualified healthcare practitioner.

Vitamin A and vitamin B complex with extra biotin, PABA, inositol, and pantothenic acid can increase hair growth and health. Mineral deficiencies, especially of iron, silicon, and zinc, can contribute to hair loss. All amino acids are essential to healthy hair because hair is nearly 98 percent protein. Essential fatty acids strengthen and nourish the hair – excellent sources are evening primrose oil and black currant seed oil. Lecithin, an emulsifier, is valuable in the assimilation of dietary fats. Some foods found to be helpful for healthy hair are grains, nuts, seeds, rice bran syrup, fruits, vegetables, and fish.

Many individual herbs and botanicals are believed to be useful in keeping hair healthy. Alfalfa, sarsaparilla, and black cohosh are believed to help to balance hormones. Licorice helps the adrenal glands, while horsetail, jojoba, blessed thistle, dulse, kelp, and comfrey are rich in minerals. Other herbs used to benefit the hair are red clover, rosemary, parsley, oatstraw, red raspberry, watercress, wormwood, sage, pau d'arco, yarrow, and slippery elm.

I have seen dramatic improvement in the hair of many people who supplement their diets with vitamins and herbs. Results often take months, so persistence and patience are necessary.

MAKING NATURAL HAIR CARE PRODUCTS

This section contains recipes for shampoos, rinses, and conditioners made with herbs or other natural products. Some recipes are for specific hair types (fine, medium, or coarse textures) as well as for dry, normal, or oily hair. Natural, homemade hair care products are inexpensive to make and are better for the environment because they are biodegradable and there's not a lot of packaging to dispose of. And be aware that a number of commercial products contain petroleum byproducts, which have a tendency to build up on the hair.

Many of the ingredients for these recipes are easily available food items, such as eggs, fruits, olive oil, and lemons. Others, such as herbs and essential oils, can be found at health food stores and drug stores.

All products should be stored in glass or plastic containers and kept in a cool, dark, dry place. Products containing fresh ingredients such as dairy products and fruit should be kept in the refrigerator.

See shampoo recipes below and on page 14.

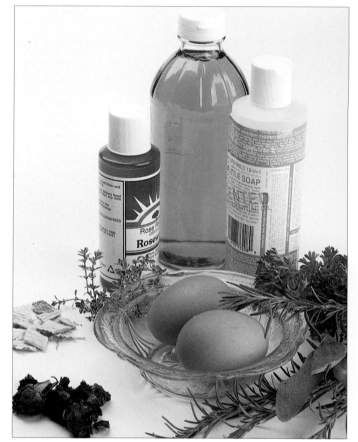

Pictured above: Shampoo Supplies

SHAMPOO RECIPES

Soapwort Shampoo

A gentle herbal shampoo for dry or normal hair.

Ingredients:

1/2 cup crushed soapwort root and leaves

8 cups distilled water

Over medium heat, gently steep water and soapwort root and leaves in a large glass or stainless steel saucepan for 15 minutes. Strain and store in a bottle.

Egg Shampoo

A protein boost for any type of hair.

Ingredients:

1 egg

Crack egg into bowl. Beat lightly. Use half the mixture to shampoo hair. Rinse with lukewarm water. Repeat. Finish with Lemon Rinse. (See the section on rinses.)

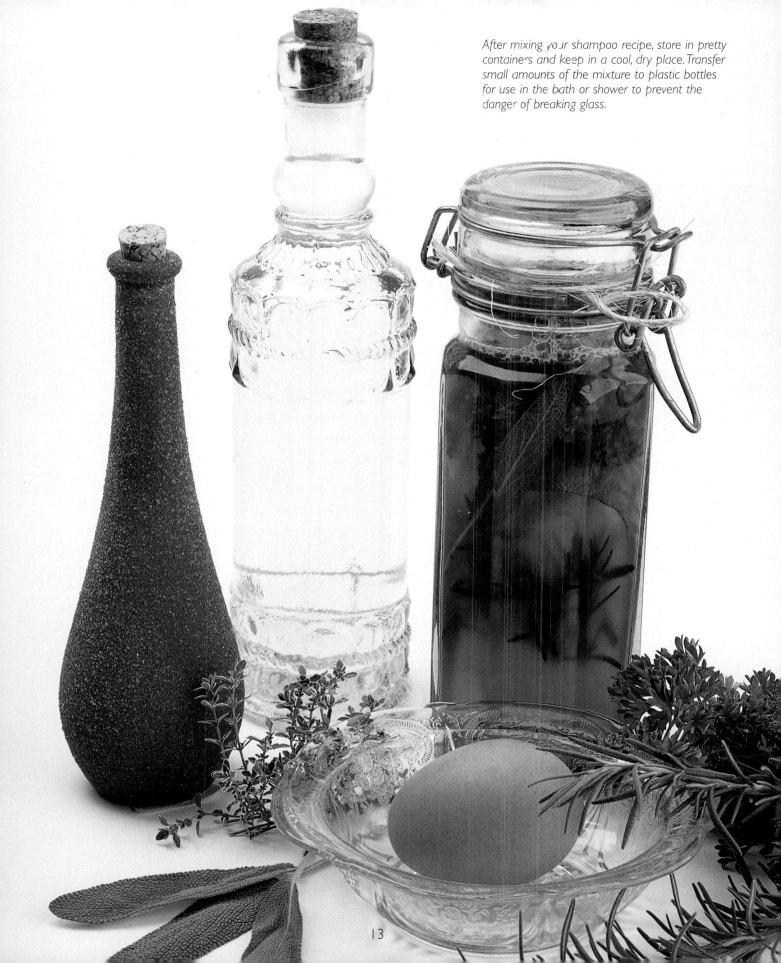

After mixing your shampoo recipe, store in pretty containers and keep in a cool, dry place. Transfer small amounts of the mixture to plastic bottles for use in the bath or shower to prevent the danger of breaking glass.

13

SHAMPOO RECIPES

Rosewater Shampoo
Especially good for fine, limp hair.

Ingredients:

4 tablespoons rosewater

4 tablespoons apple cider vinegar

4 raw eggs

Place all ingredients in a bowl and whisk together. Use liberally. Leave in the hair 10 minutes for extra conditioning before rinsing. Store in the refrigerator no longer than 1 week.

Four Herb Shampoo
For use on all hair types.

Ingredients:

2 tablespoons fresh parsley

2 tablespoons rosemary leaves

2 tablespoons sage leaves

2 tablespoons thyme leaves

1 cup boiling water

1 cup mild liquid soap, such as a castile soap

Add herbs to boiling water. Remove from heat. Cover. Let steep 20 minutes. Add soap. Strain into a container. Let stand overnight before using.

CONDITIONER RECIPES

Mayonnaise Hair Pack

Ingredients:

1 cup natural (not lite) mayonnaise

Apply a generous amount to freshly shampooed, towel dried hair. Place a plastic bag over the hair (but **not** over the entire head) and leave on for at least 30 minutes. Remove plastic bag and shampoo normally.

Olive Oil Conditioner
This conditioner will improve the strength and shine of the hair.

Ingredients:

1 cup of olive oil

10 drops of your favorite essential oil

(My favorites are rose and lavender.)

Mix oils. Let sit for at least 24 hours. Apply a tablespoon of warm oil to freshly shampooed hair. Leave for 20 to 30 minutes.

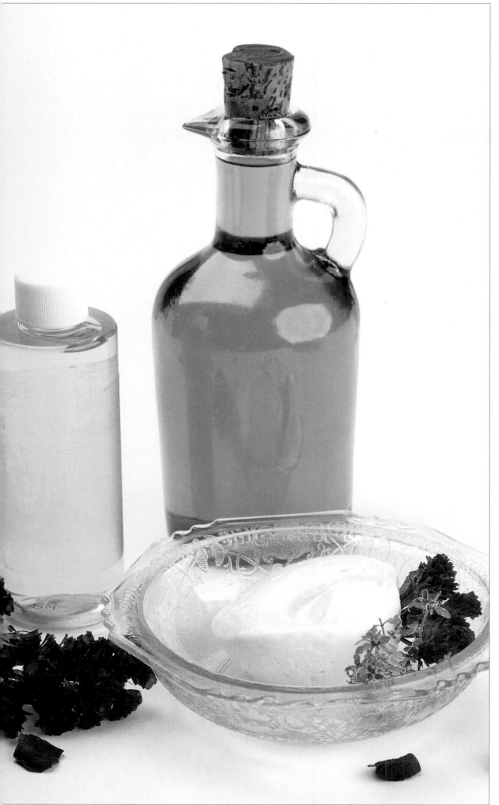

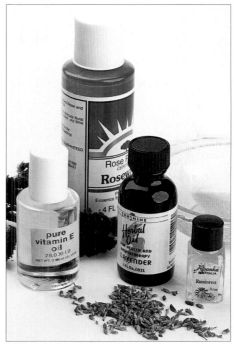

Pictured above: Supplies for making conditioners

Jojoba Conditioner

Especially good for dry, coarse-textured hair.

Ingredients:

1 cup rosewater

1 tablespoon jojoba oil

10 drops vitamin E oil

Warm water gently in a double boiler. When hot, add jojoba oil. Whisk in vitamin E oil and blend well. Apply to clean hair and leave on for at least 10 minutes.

Pictured above: Conditioners to strengthen and brighten hair.

HAIR TREATMENT RECIPES

Coconut Oil Treatment
This versatile oil can be used daily as a moisturizer.

Ingredients:

Coconut oil

Take 1/4 to 1/2 teaspoon coconut oil in the palm of one hand. Rub hands together to distribute and apply to the scalp. Massage through the ends of the hair.

Hot Oil Treatment

Ingredients:

1 oz. olive oil

Apply olive oil to shampooed, towel dried hair. Place plastic wrap or a plastic bag over the hair (but **not** over the whole head). For added benefit, apply a warm towel to the head or sit in the sun for 10 minutes. Shampoo several times to remove excess oil.

Avocado Moisturizer

Ingredients:

1 ripe avocado

Mash avocado in a bowl or puree in a blender. Apply to clean, wet hair. Leave on for 20 to 30 minutes. Rinse thoroughly.

Silky Smooth Hair Therapy
For silky hair that smells delightful.

Ingredients:

9 drops lavender essential oil

5 drops lemon grass essential oil

4 drops rosemary essential oil

1 cup jojoba oil

Combine essential oils and jojoba oil. Store in an airtight glass container. **To use:** Heat 2 tablespoons and massage into the hair. Wrap hair **but not the head** in plastic for 30 minutes.

Hair Pomade
For moisturizing.

Ingredients:

1 cup olive oil

1/2 cup beeswax

1 tablespoon coconut oil

Melt ingredients over low heat. Pour in heatproof container. Ingredients will harden in about 25 minutes. **To use:** Place a pea-sized amount of the pomade in the palm of one hand. Rub your hands together to distribute the pomade and rub lightly into the ends of the hair.

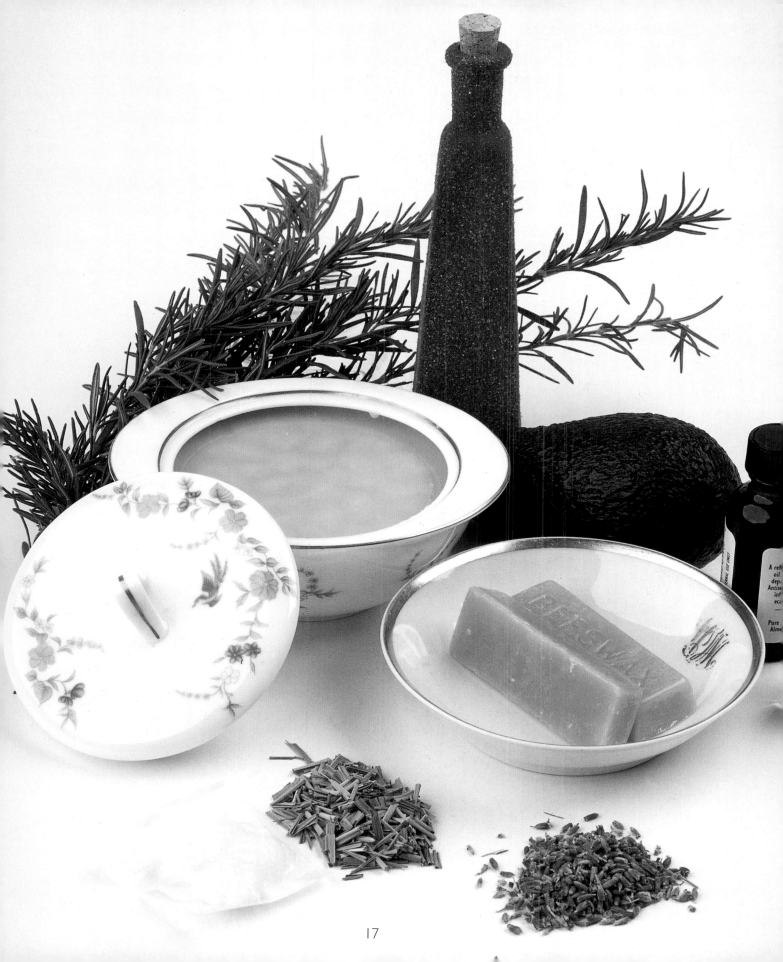

HAIR RINSE RECIPES

Vinegar Rinse

To clarify and give hair added shine.

Ingredients:

1/4 cup apple cider vinegar

2 cups distilled water

Mix ingredients and apply to shampooed hair.

Baking Soda Rinse

For clarifying. Use regularly to remove environmental pollutants, shampoo and conditioner residues, and chemical buildup. (It's great for swimmers!)

Ingredients:

1 tablespoon baking soda

1 cup distilled water

Mix ingredients. Pour through shampooed hair.

Lemon Rinse

Ingredients:

1/2 lemon

2 cups distilled water

Squeeze lemon in water. Pour through clean, towel dried hair.

Apple Cider Vinegar & Watercress Rinse

For oily hair.

Ingredients:

1 cup distilled water

2 teaspoons apple cider vinegar

2 cups watercress

Warm the water and vinegar in a saucepan. In a blender container, blend watercress with the water and vinegar mixture for 2 minutes. Strain. **To use:** Apply to shampooed hair and leave on for 10 minutes. Rinse with clear water.

Herbal Rinses

Use for fresh highlights on clean, shampooed hair.

Ingredients:

For blondes: 1/4 cup dried chamomile flowers

For redheads: 1/4 cup dried calendula petals

For brunettes: 1/4 cup dried rosemary

Distilled water

Place herbs appropriate to your hair color in a saucepan with 1 cup water. Bring to a boil. Remove from heat and let steep 30 minutes. Strain and refrigerate. *To use:* Apply to clean hair.

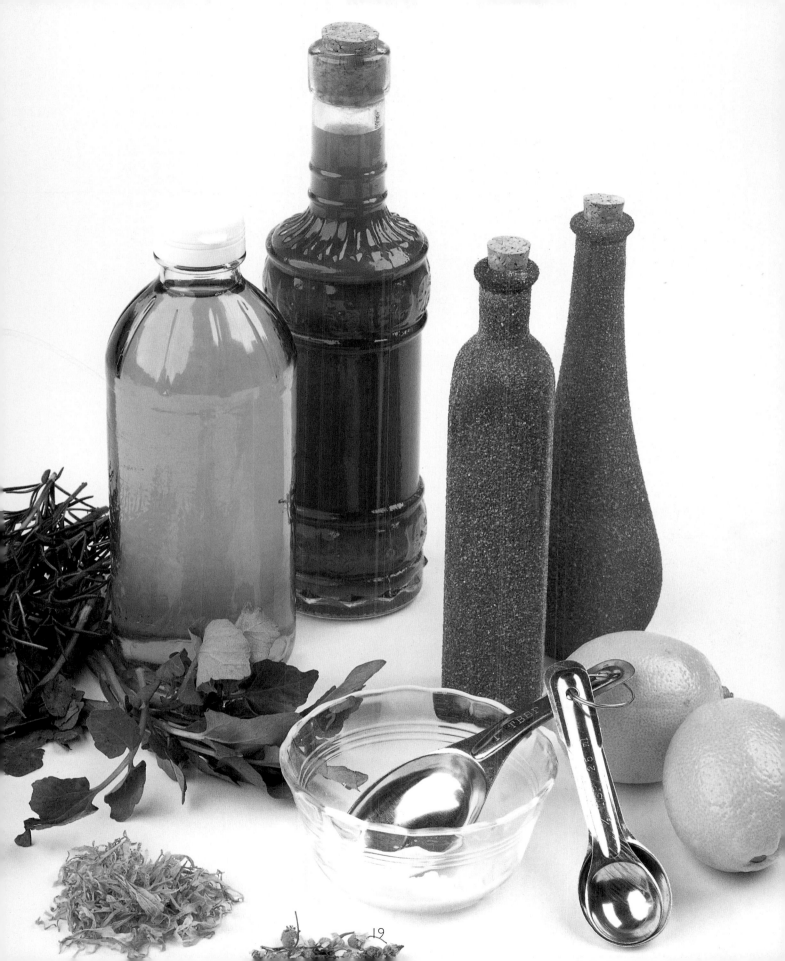

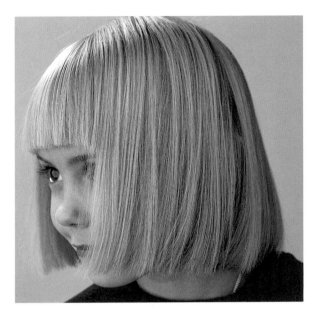

Choosing a Style

Hair texture and bone structure determine what kinds of styles can be worn effectively. Other factors to consider are lifestyle and face shape. It's important to talk with the person whose hair you will be cutting, to ask the person about preferences regarding style and length, and to develop your skills as an observer. Studying faces and hair texture is fascinating. The following pages explore these topics.

HAIR TYPES, TEXTURE, AND DENSITY

It's important to identify the texture, the type, and the density of the hair before beginning the cut. Any of the hair forms can be fine, medium, or coarse in texture.

✄ Hair Types

Straight hair comes out of a round follicle, a tiny tube in the scalp from which the hair grows. This type of hair tends to grow from the scalp at a slight angle so that it lays against the head more than other types.

Wavy hair has a little more body and is more easily styled.

Curly hair grows out of a nearly flat follicle and tends to grow up and out from the scalp. That is why curly hair may look thicker than straight hair, which might not be the case. Curly hair can be fine as well as coarse.

Super curly hair comes out of a flat follicle and grows from the scalp at the greatest angle – straight up.

✄ Texture

You must observe and feel the hair to recognize and understand hair texture. The texture is determined by the size of the hair shaft. There are three major textures: fine, medium, and coarse.

Fine hair is soft and shiny and often goes limp or flat. Very fine, thin hair usually does best when left one length although if the person's bone structure is especially delicate, a more layered, spikier cut can be worn.

Medium textured hair is stronger, feels thicker, and holds its shape well. Medium textured hair is more versatile, allowing the person's bone structure to determine the style. If the ends of the hair feel coarse and dry, conditioning is required.

Coarse hair is dry, bulky, and wiry and lacks shine. Rich conditioning is required, and controlling the bulk with the proper cut is important. Coarse textured hair usually looks best layered but is ideal if a very full look is desired.

✄ Hair Density

This refers to the number of hairs growing out of the scalp per square inch. We usually refer to the density as having **thin hair** or **thick hair**. With thin hair, the scalp can be seen when the hair is wet and when conditioned, the hair seems flat. If the hair is thick, it seems busy and needs bulk cut out of it to control it. Coarse textured hair tends to be bulky or thick. Dense hair looks best in a cut that is layered with the volume reduced. Thin hair that is also fine looks best with a blunt cut so that it appears thicker.

LIFESTYLE FACTORS

Most people want a cut that works well with their hair and is easy to care for. To find the best style, get to know the people's lifestyles and their daily habits concerning their hair. How often do they shampoo? How much time do they have to devote every day to hair care? What about their occupation or leisure activities (sports, hobbies, etc.)? A student on the swim team or someone who swims for exercise may want a short, quick-drying style; an aspiring ballerina may relish the idea of long locks that can be worn up or pulled back.

A proper cut can save precious time for most people. To help cope with the hustle and bustle of modern life, many people want wash-and-wear hair – a style that doesn't require blow drying – or hair that falls into place without a lot of fussing.

BONE STRUCTURE

My rule of thumb is the more delicate the facial bone structure, the shorter the hair can be worn. People with more chiseled features and larger bone structure usually need more hair. But do listen to how people feel – if they want hair that overpowers the face – well, even someone with delicate bone structure can wear lots of full hair successfully.

FACE SHAPES

The cut should be flattering to the shape of the person's face. Identifying the shape of the face is an important part of choosing a style. Most heads are round to oval. Feel the head so you will become familiar with the shape that you will be sculpting. To feel the shape of the skull, put your hands in the person's hair and feel the bone structure under the scalp with your hands. Don't be timid – this is an important part of developing your skills.

To determine a face shape, first measure the face with a ruler or tape measure. Write the measurements down so that you can refer to them. a) Measure across the top of the cheekbones. b) Measure across jaw line. c) Measure across the widest part of the forehead. d) Measure from the top of the head to the point of chin.

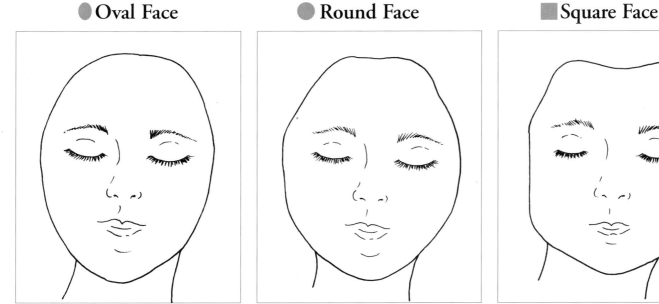

● Oval Face

If you have this face shape, the length is equal to 1-1/2 times the width. Oval-shaped faces look good with almost any style, so let the texture of the hair determine what looks best.

● Round Face

A round face is as wide as it is long. A round face looks best with a cut that creates the illusion of a longer, thinner face. You don't want to give a round-faced person a chin-length blunt cut because it will make the face look very round. If the hair is very straight, a shoulder length blunt cut will work. Layering the hair – either long or short – is usually best because this creates more height on the top. Light, layered bangs worn off the forehead are usually best.

■ Square Face

With a square face, the forehead, jaw line and cheekbones are nearly equal in width. Both round and square faces can wear similar cuts. A square face needs a cut that softens the jaw line to create an illusion of length. Cutting long layers with soft curls around the chin looks nice. Softening the hairline with bangs also looks good.

🔘 Oblong Face

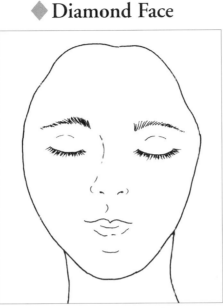

This face is longer than it is wide. The oblong face needs a cut that creates the illusion of width and shortens the length. A chin-length blunt cut works well. Bangs create width and make the face look shorter.

🔶 Diamond Face

The jawbone and forehead is narrow, with the cheekbones being wider. The diamond-shaped face looks great with bangs. Soft curls that are shoulder length work nicely. The chin line needs fullness to fill in the narrowness of the chin.

💜 Heart Face

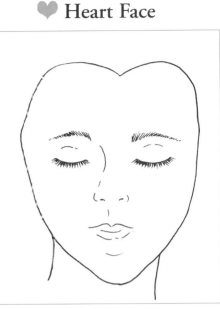

This face is wide at the forehead and cheekbones, and narrow at the jawline. A soft layered style with bangs and length with fullness in the back is appropriate.

🔺 Pear or Triangle Shape

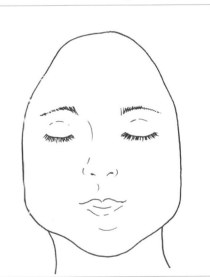

The pear-shaped face has a small forehead and a heavy or square chin. The forehead measurement is smaller than the jawline measurement. Hair that is shoulder length and feathered toward the chin and neck and worn away from the face is best.

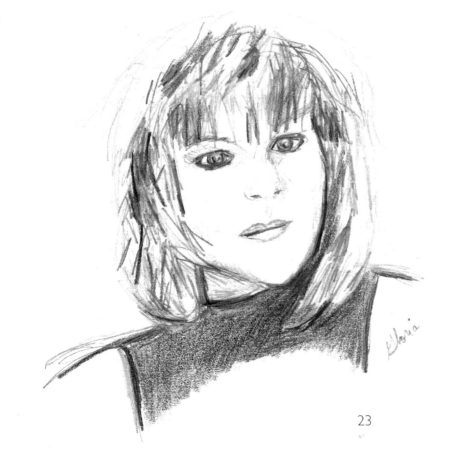

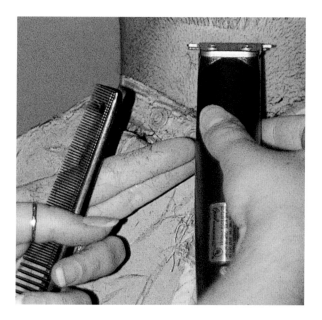

HAIRCUTTING

Tools & Equipment

It's very important to have the proper tools and equipment.
You can buy them at beauty supply stores. Prices will vary.

Pictured at right — clockwise from top: Hair brush, butterfly clips,
clippers, scissors, scissors case, and comb.

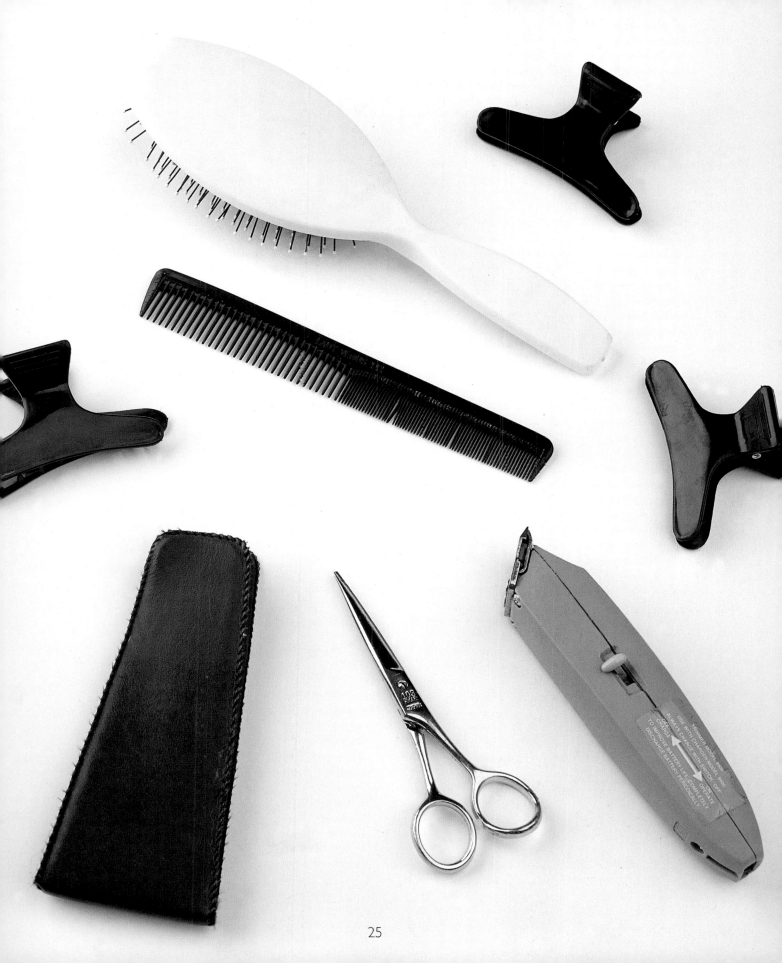

✀ Scissors

Scissors are your most important tool. Make sure they are sharp, feel comfortable to hold, and fit your hand well. A serviceable pair will cost $25 to $30; a good pair can cost several hundred dollars. The best scissors are made of steel. They can be purchased at department stores, cutlery shops, or beauty supply stores.

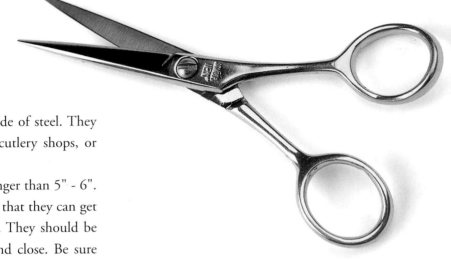

Choose a pair of scissors that are no longer than 5" - 6". The blades should be sleek and narrow so that they can get into tight places such as around the ears. They should be comfortable to hold and easy to open and close. Be sure that they are sharp.

Take care of your scissors and they will stay sharp and last for years. Dry the blades after each haircut, wiping off all pieces of hair. Dropping scissors could break the point and mis-align the blades.

✀ Comb

A comb is used in conjunction with the scissors when cutting the hair. A comb that glides easily through the hair and fits your hand well will become your scissors' best friend. Combs can be purchased for a couple of dollars. Try to find one with inches marked on it. Choose a hard, sturdy, yet thin comb with the teeth spaced at two different widths. The wider spaced side is used to comb the hair when wet so that the hair is not stretched. The narrow spaced side is used to smooth the hair sections for cutting.

✀ Hair Brush

I like a paddle brush for brushing out tangles. The bristles can be wire, synthetic, or natural. This is used for styling the hair when blow drying.

✀ Hair Clips

Four large butterfly clips are needed for securing sections of hair during cutting. These can be purchased for a few dollars. These type of clips can hold a lot of hair and they won't slip.

✀ Cape & Towel

A plastic haircutting cape is a good professional touch, and it keeps cut hair and dripping water off clothes. You can purchase one at a store that sells beauty supplies. A towel is needed to blot hair after shampooing or wetting, and a dry towel can be wrapped around the shoulders if a cape is not available.

✀ Spray Bottle

A plastic water spray bottle is used to keep the hair damp when cutting, not dripping wet. Spray the hair then comb through it to dampen. Choose one that's comfortable to hold and use with one hand.

✀ Clippers

Optional:

A pair of clippers – also called trimmers – are not necessary for all cuts. You'll want them for short, head-hugging styles and for trimming around the neck and sideburns for shorter cuts.

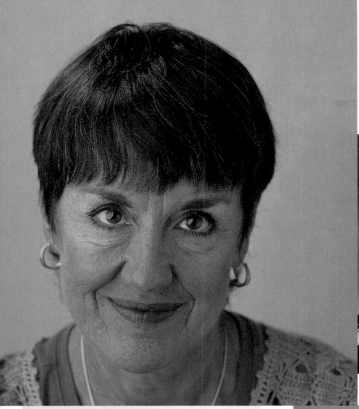

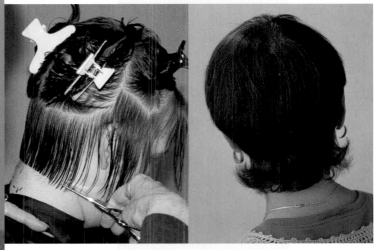

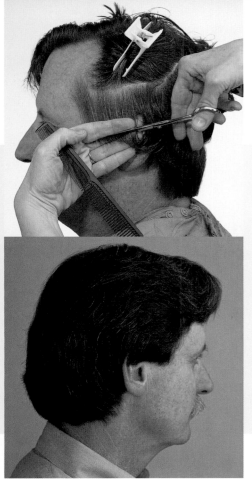

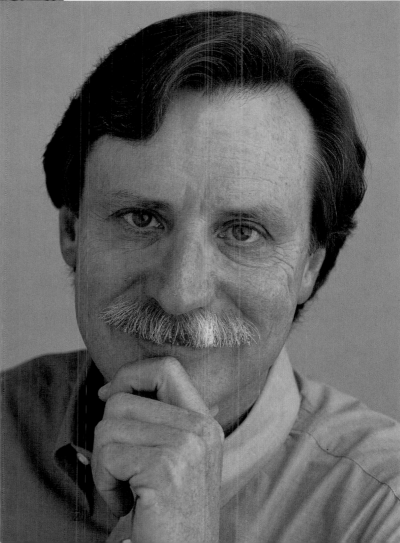

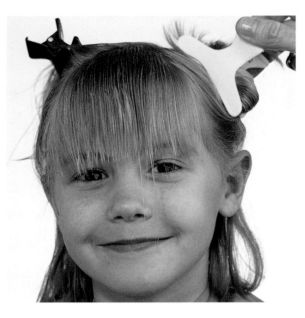

Preparation

Cutting hair is an opportunity to make your friend, partner, or child feel pampered. Touch is a powerful tool. Touching the head and cutting the hair are rituals that have been passed down through the ages. The effects can be healing and beautifying or uncomfortable and disastrous.

✂ Preparing Yourself

The atmosphere of the haircut is affected by how relaxed and comfortable you are. Take a moment to relax before beginning the actual cutting. Sitting quietly, clearing your mind of as much clutter as possible, and centering yourself help open you to the creative process. Try lighting a scented candle or incense. Lavender fragrance has a calming effect.

✂ Preparing the Environment

Be sure to consider the environment for haircutting. Choose an area where you will have plenty of room and that can be swept easily. A quiet environment without distractions is essential for proper concentration. Listening to relaxing music, such as classical, new age, or soft rock, is often helpful and enjoyable.

Good lighting and a stool at the proper height are crucial. A room with natural light is best, but any well-lit room will do. A stool should be used so you can move around freely; working at eye level is most efficient. Have a table handy to keep your tools on.

✂ Preparing the Person Receiving the Cut

Make sure the person getting the haircut is relaxed and as comfortable as possible when you begin. A cape or covering such as a sheet or towel to keep the cut hair off clothing is nice. Massaging the scalp and neck and gently brushing the hair can have a relaxing effect.

Communicating verbally affects the comfort level of both the hair cutter and the person getting a haircut. Talk about hair texture and bone structure. Agree on the style and how much hair is going to be removed. (Looking at photographs can be helpful.) This is when a comb marked with inches becomes a truly useful tool. When someone says, "Cut off one inch of hair," you can use the markings on the comb to make sure you both have the same visual concept of exactly what "one inch" looks like.

✂ Hair Preparation for Cutting

The hair should be shampooed and towel dried for cutting. Hair is easiest to cut when it is kept wet, so have a spray bottle of water handy.

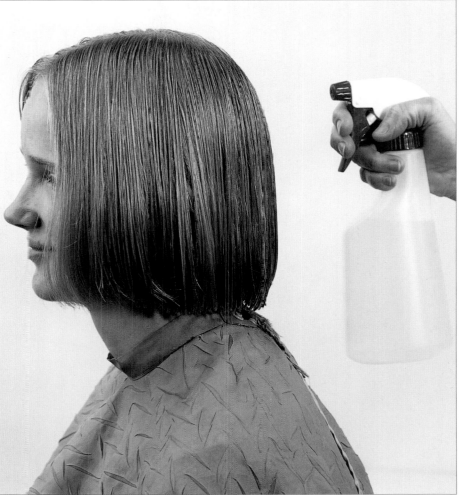

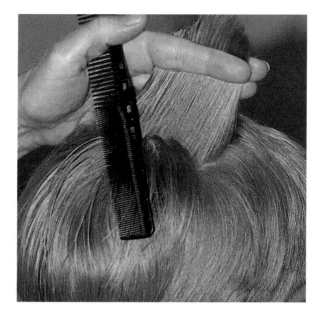

Techniques for Cutting Hair

I'm going to let you in on some tricks of the trade.
Once your know the proper way to hold the comb and
scissors, the process will be much easier. Also, there is a
system I use for cutting hair, and I follow that same system,
no matter how long or short the hair. When you learn my
system of establishing your guidelines, then you will be able
to cut any length hair.

HOLDING THE SCISSORS & COMB

Being able to work with scissors in one hand and comb in the other is the basic skill needed for a good cut. It takes practice, so don't get discouraged if it feels awkward to begin with.

Here's an exercise for developing the proper scissors technique: Hold the scissors in your hand and place the lower blade on a table or hard surface, then open and close the blades of the scissors. The lower blade will be stable while the upper blade moves. That's what you want to happen when you cut – you want the lower blade stable.

Practice moving the comb from hand to hand, as that is what you will do while you're cutting. If you're like most people, you'll section and comb the hair with your dominant hand, then move the comb to your non-dominant hand as you cut with your dominant hand. Again, practice makes perfect! Don't give up if it's not comfortable right away.

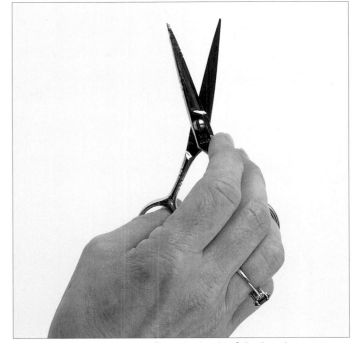

Holding the scissors – view from the back of the hand.

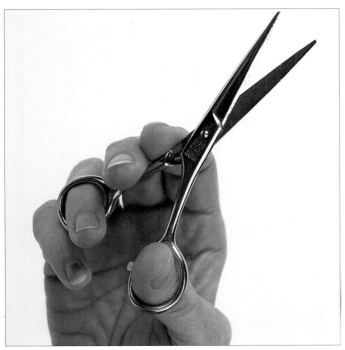

Holding the scissors – view from the palm.

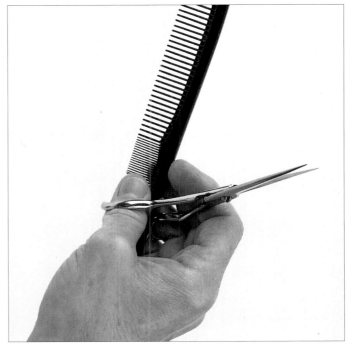

Holding the comb while holding the scissors.

HAIRCUTTING ANGLES

Angles are measured in degrees. To cut, you will form an angle with the scalp and the hair. Know that whichever angle you are cutting the hair from, gravity pulls it down. Try to visualize how the hair will fall.

The separation between the scalp and the hair can be measured by the degrees of the angle. You will be working with 180, 90 and 45 degree angles, which are also called elevations. A 90 degree angle is when the hair comes straight out from the head. A 180 degree angle is straight up. A 45 degree angle is half of a 90 degree angle. Practice holding hair at these angles. Eventually that will become second nature as a cutting skill.

The angle the hair is held when cutting determines whether the style will be long or short layered. Holding the hair at a 90-degree angle will result in each hair being the same length, creating a short layered style. Holding the hair at a 45-degree angle will result in long layers. Holding the hair at 180-degrees will give the most drastic layers.

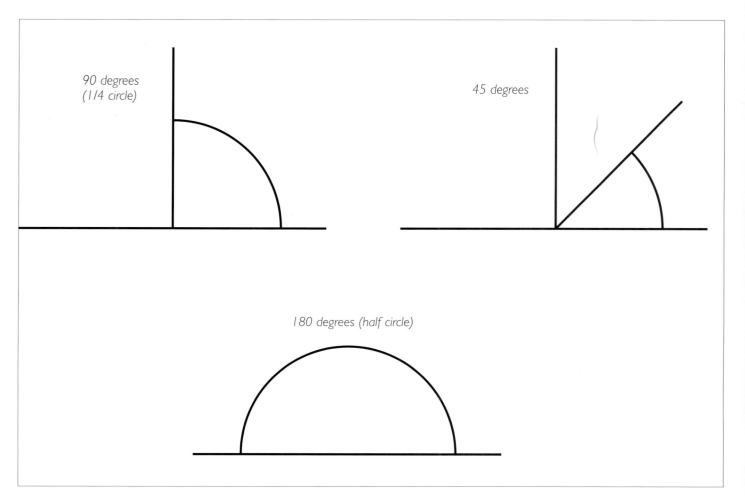

90 degrees
(1/4 circle)

45 degrees

180 degrees (half circle)

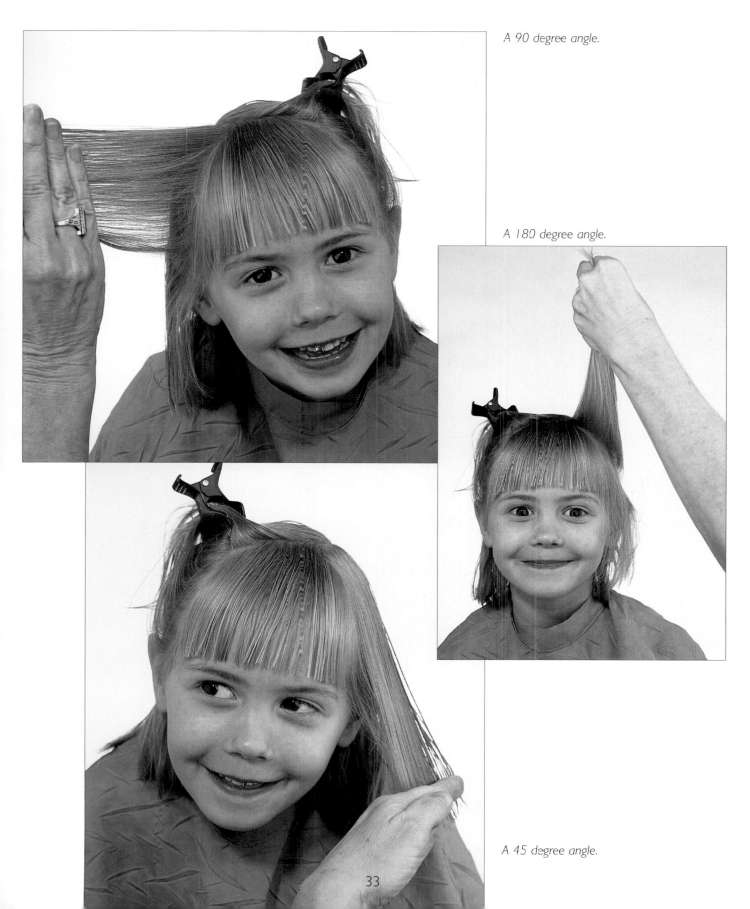

A 90 degree angle.

A 180 degree angle.

A 45 degree angle.

33

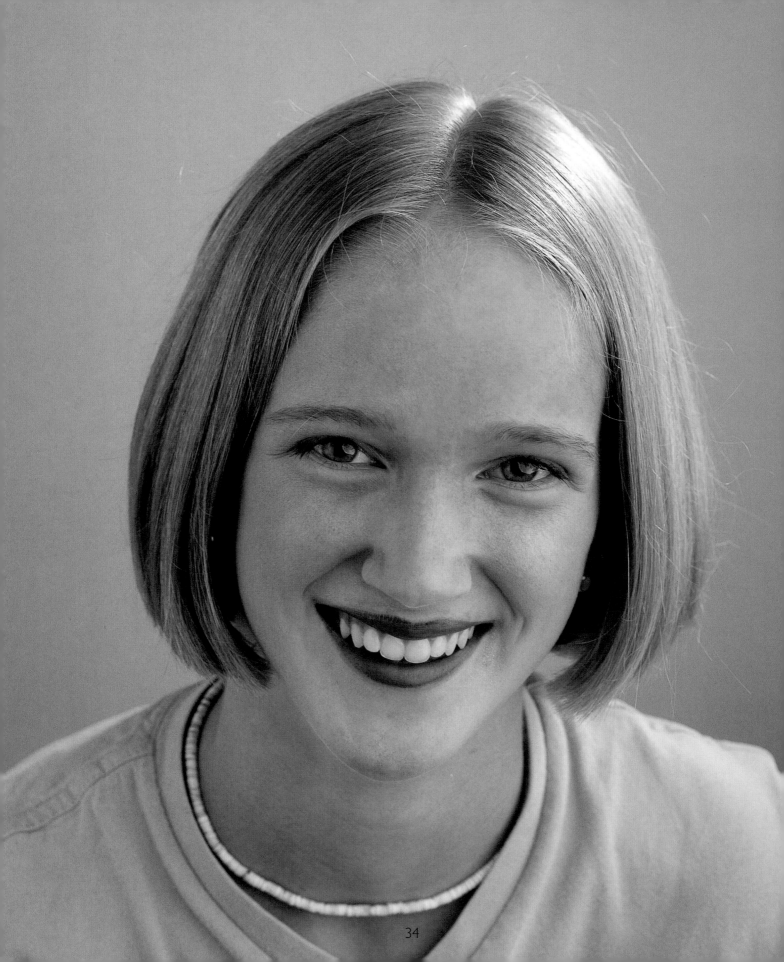

ESTABLISHING GUIDES

Establishing guides are the key to a successful haircut. Guides, which are also called guidelines, will keep you on the correct cutting path – they are the pattern you will cut by. Cut these to the length you wish the hair to be. After the guides have been established, they should not be cut into or altered. The guides for the back, sides, and front are cut from a 1" section of hair around the entire perimeter of the head. The shape and length of the guide depends on the haircut you are doing. The guides are used for both one-length cuts and layered cuts.

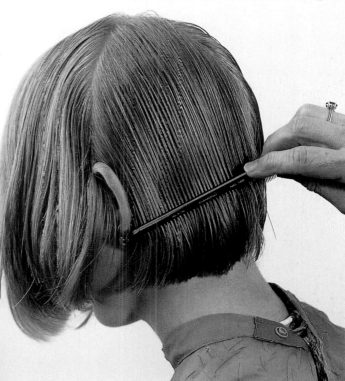

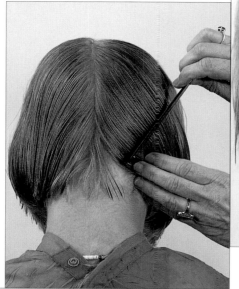

1

Part wet hair, if it is long enough, from the center of the forehead to the center of the nape of the neck.

2 Then part hair from ear to ear.

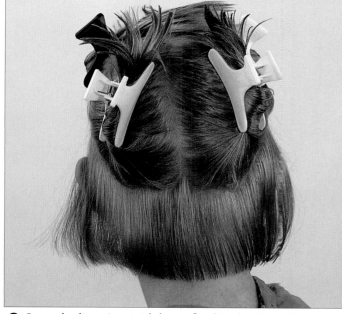

3 Secure back sections with butterfly clips, leaving a 1" section at the bottom for the guide.

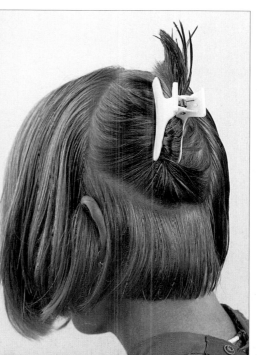

4

A back view of sectioned and clipped hair.

continued on next page

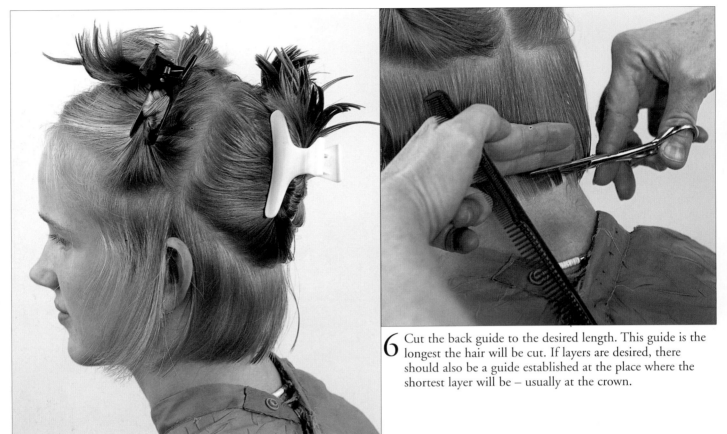

6 Cut the back guide to the desired length. This guide is the longest the hair will be cut. If layers are desired, there should also be a guide established at the place where the shortest layer will be – usually at the crown.

5 All hair is butterfly clipped and ready to be cut.

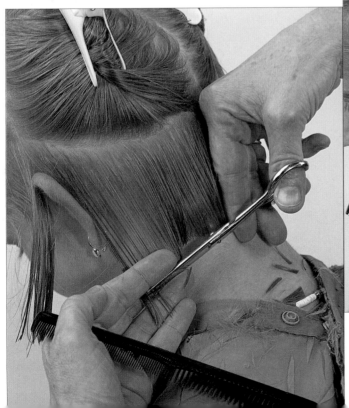

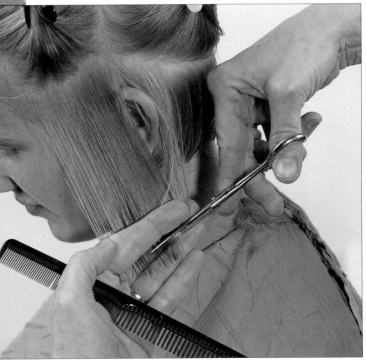

7 Continue to cut the guide in the back, moving around to the side.

8 Cut the side guide to the desired length.

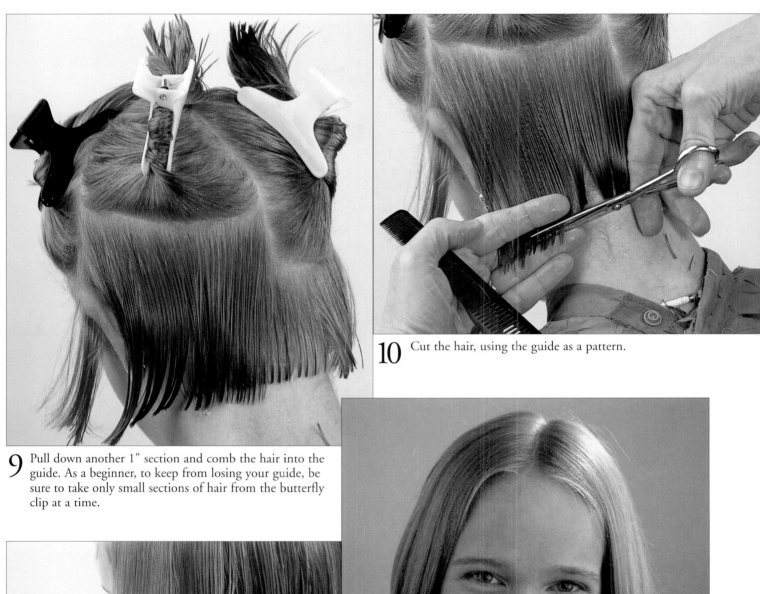

9 Pull down another 1" section and comb the hair into the guide. As a beginner, to keep from losing your guide, be sure to take only small sections of hair from the butterfly clip at a time.

10 Cut the hair, using the guide as a pattern.

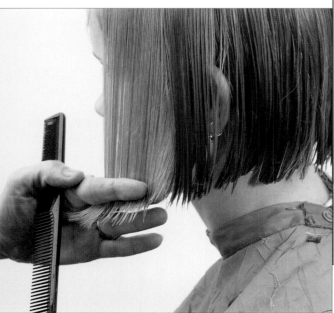

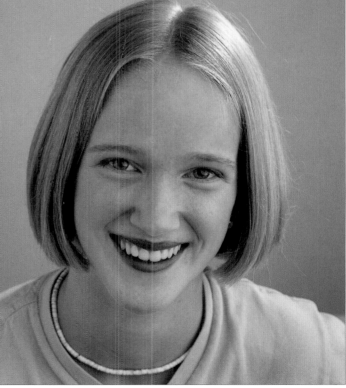

11 Continue to pull sections from the clips. Comb the hair into the guide, then cut.

12 The finished cut.

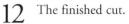

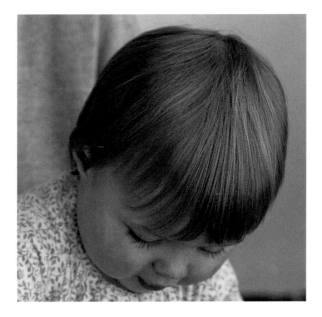

Children's
HAIRCUTTING
Styles

Children's cuts should be kept simple. Most children have fine hair until puberty, and fine hair can be a challenge because it tangles easily. It is best to keep this fine, delicate hair short – a short cut gives the hair body and fullness and is more comfortable for the child. The ends of fine hair split easily, and frequent trimming minimizes damage. I find that trimming fine hair regularly helps the hair thicken.

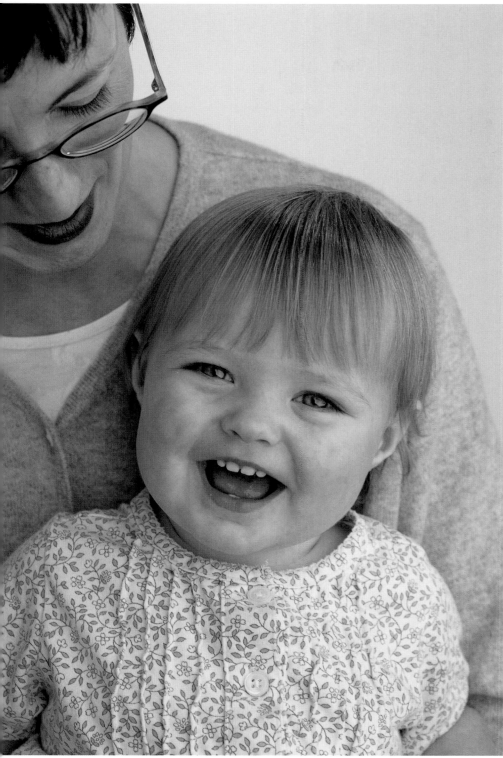

Pictured above: This baby fine hair merely needs to be trimmed at bangs. Babies move fast so have an adult hold the baby while you quickly and carefully trim bangs.

✂ Tips for Cutting Children's Hair

• Children under the age of three usually have short attention spans, so work as quickly as possible.

• Have a plan before you begin and always have another adult around for children under three years, just in case you need help distracting the child.

• Toddlers need added distractions – anything you can do to keep them still will help. A toddler may need to be held by another adult while the haircut takes place. (A baby should always be held.) Butterfly clips are always a good distraction – kids love to play with them.

• Don't worry about getting hair on the child. Usually little ones don't like to be encumbered with a hair-cutting cape. Their clothes can be taken off and shaken after the cut is finished to remove the hair.

• Try not to use the word "cut" around small children – I've found the word frightens them, so I say "trim" instead.

• All children will hate having a hair-cut if you make them sit too long – always keep this in mind.

• Older children usually can sit longer, so a more time-consuming style could be chosen. I tell older children that the time will be shorter if they can sit still – this usually works.

GIRLS' SHORT ONE-LENGTH CUT

Hair Type: Thick, fine, straight

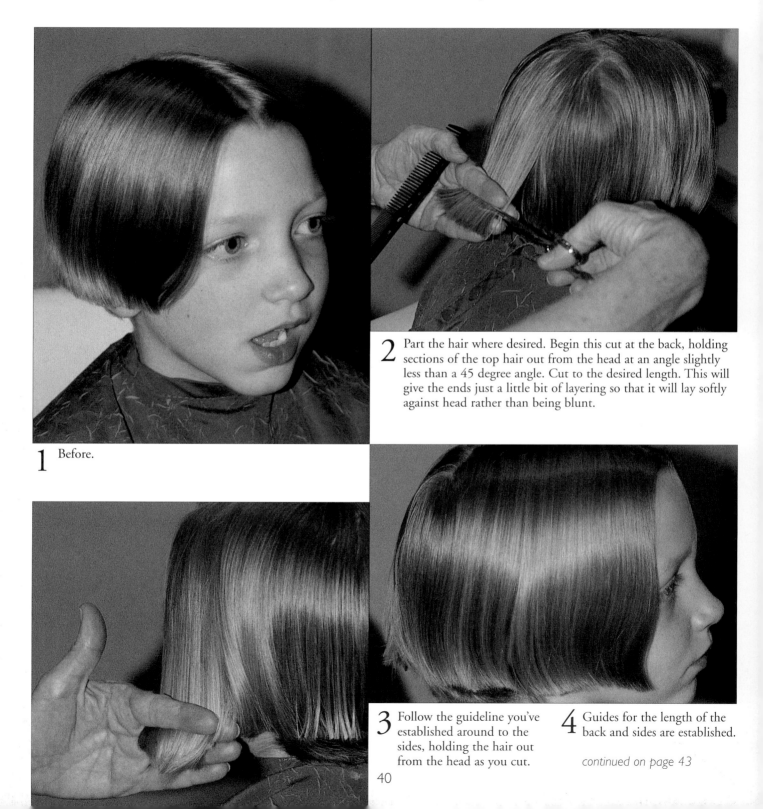

1 Before.

2 Part the hair where desired. Begin this cut at the back, holding sections of the top hair out from the head at an angle slightly less than a 45 degree angle. Cut to the desired length. This will give the ends just a little bit of layering so that it will lay softly against head rather than being blunt.

3 Follow the guideline you've established around to the sides, holding the hair out from the head as you cut.

4 Guides for the length of the back and sides are established.

continued on page 43

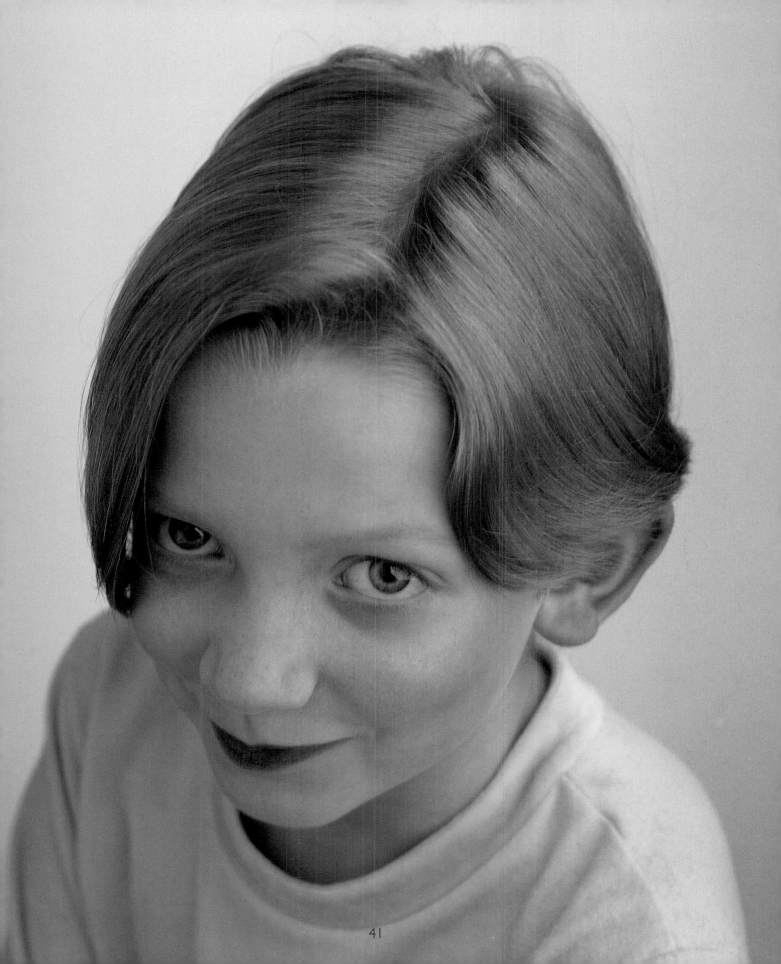

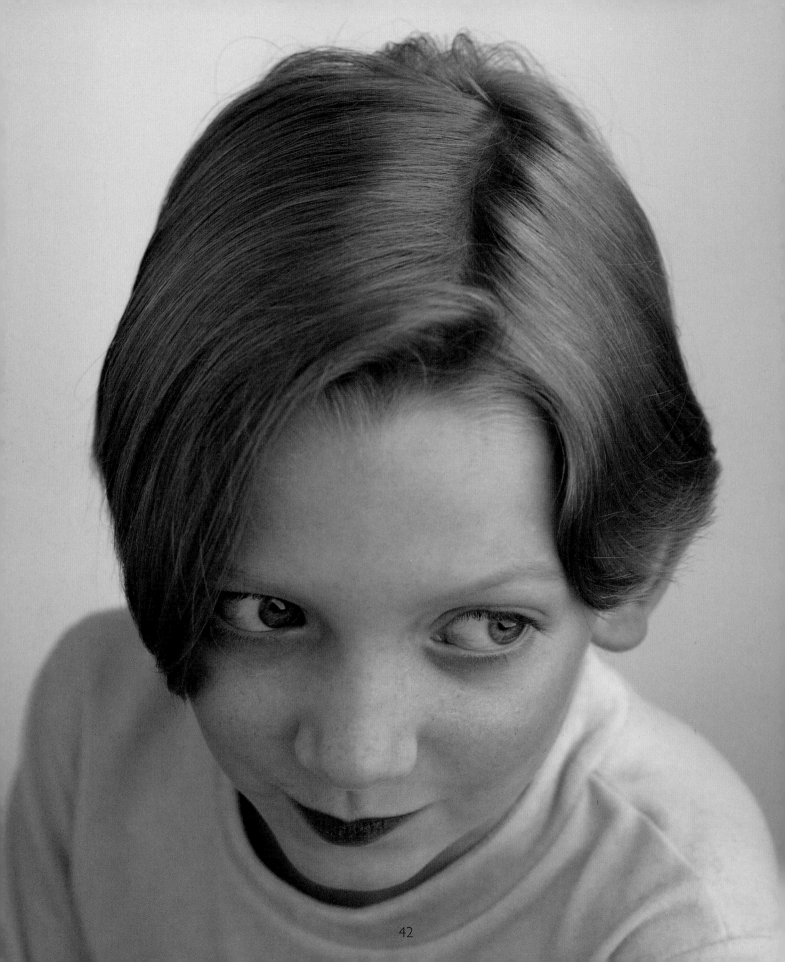

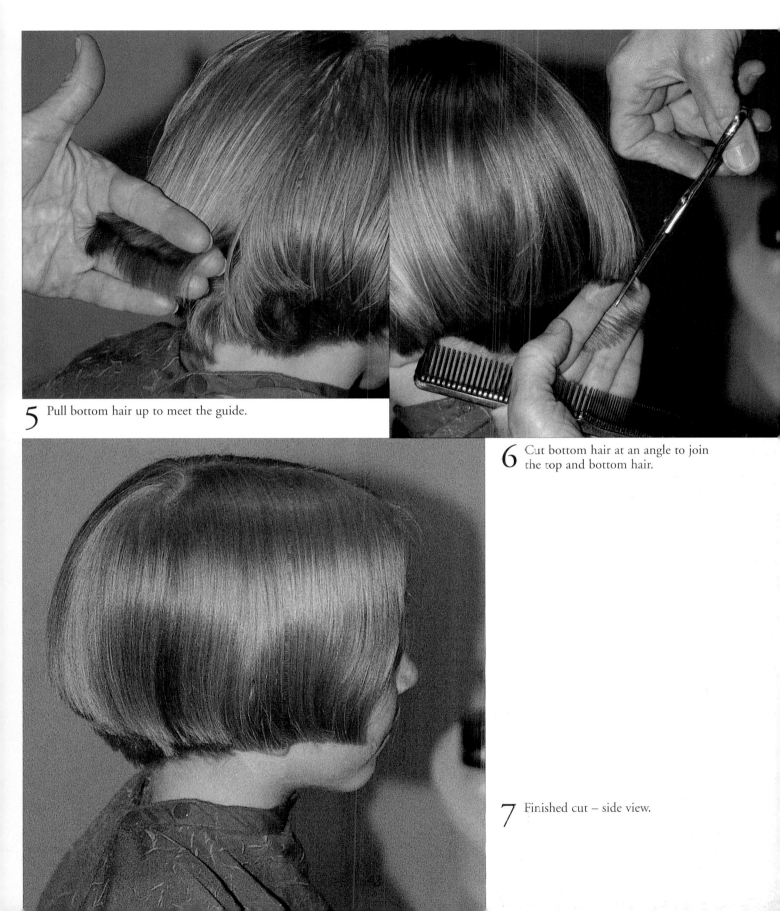

5 Pull bottom hair up to meet the guide.

6 Cut bottom hair at an angle to join the top and bottom hair.

7 Finished cut – side view.

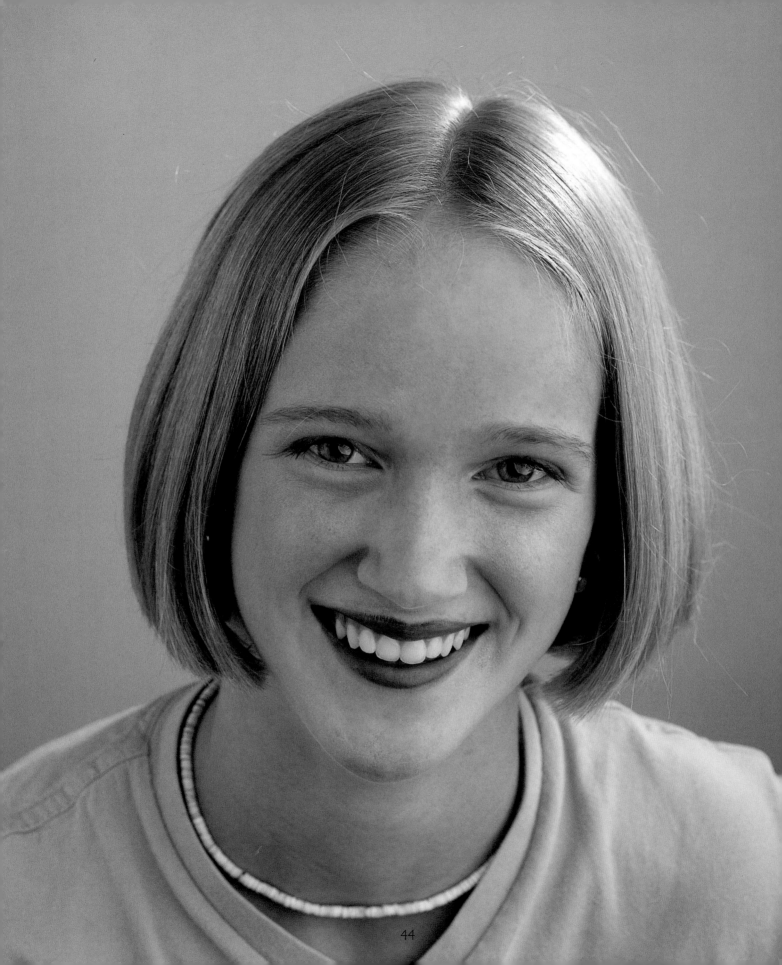

GIRLS' MEDIUM ONE-LENGTH CUT

This is a very easy cut and it looks great on any type of hair. It is easy to care for yet is a classic style that looks good on most face shapes. It is one of the best styles for straight hair.

Hair Type: Medium texture, medium thickness, straight.

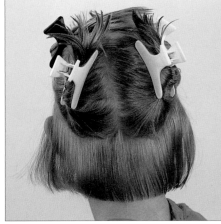

1 Section hair, leaving a 1" section at bottom to cut as a guide.

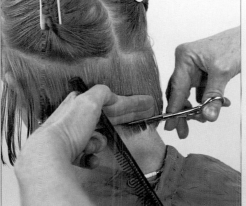

2 Cut back and sides to desired length.

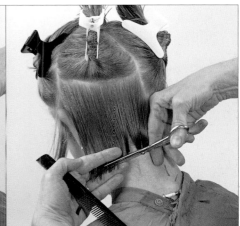

3 Be sure the head is straight and erect or you won't get an even cut. Pull 1" sections of hair down from clip and cut them the same length as the guides.

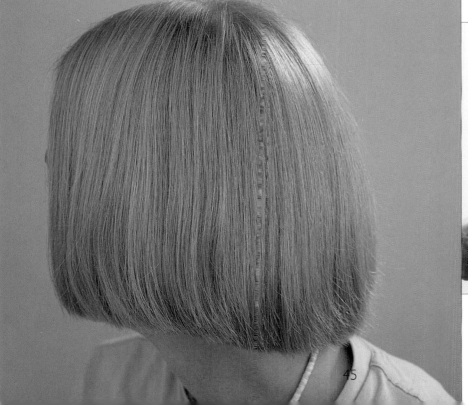

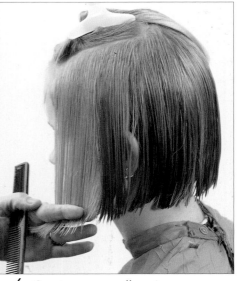

4 Continue to cut all sections even with guide.

GIRLS' MEDIUM ONE-LENGTH STYLE

This style is one-length with bangs. It is very popular with kids and parents because it is neat, and can be worn in a number of styles. It is cut in the same way as shown previously for the one-length style.

1 Comb down hair for bangs first before cutting remainder of hair. Cut bangs by holding hair out with fingers. Place end of scissors where you want length to be. Hold scissors horizontally and cut up to fingers. Do not try to use the scissors against the child's head because a sudden move could cause a wound.

2 Section hair, leaving a section at perimeter, back and sides to cut as a guide.

3 Bring hair down in sections and cut even with guides.

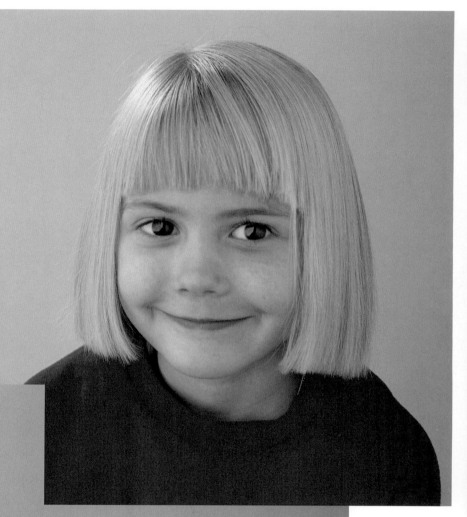

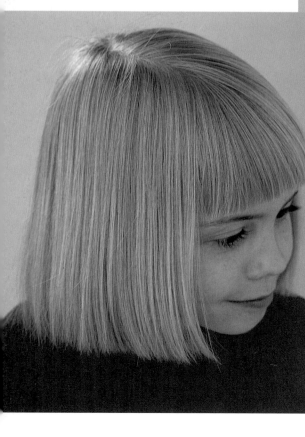

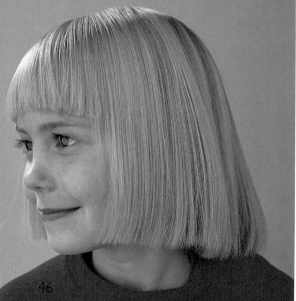

LONG ONE-LENGTH CUT

The one-length cut is great for any age or hair type as you can see. This cut was created like the previous one-length cuts, with the sides being cut at an angle to be shorter as the hair gets closer to the front. When the sides were cut, they were pulled out from the head at a slight angle to subtly layer them. This helps to frame the face nicely. Before cutting, part the hair where desired.

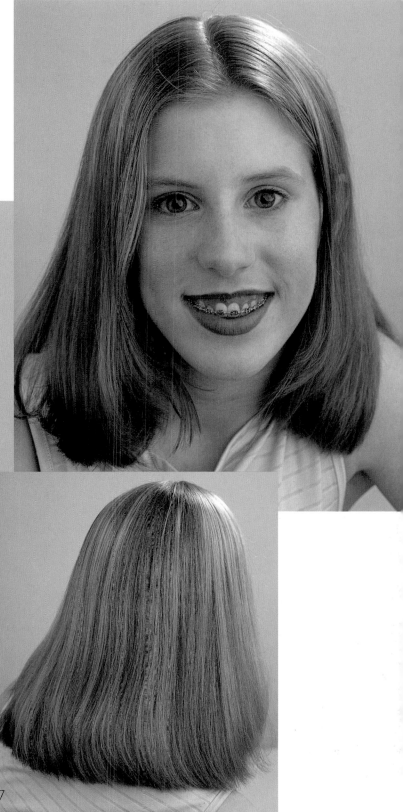

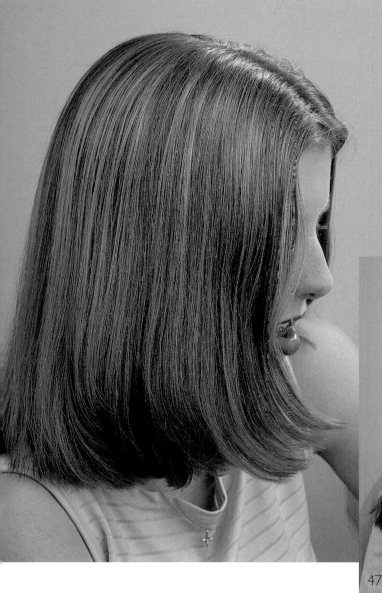

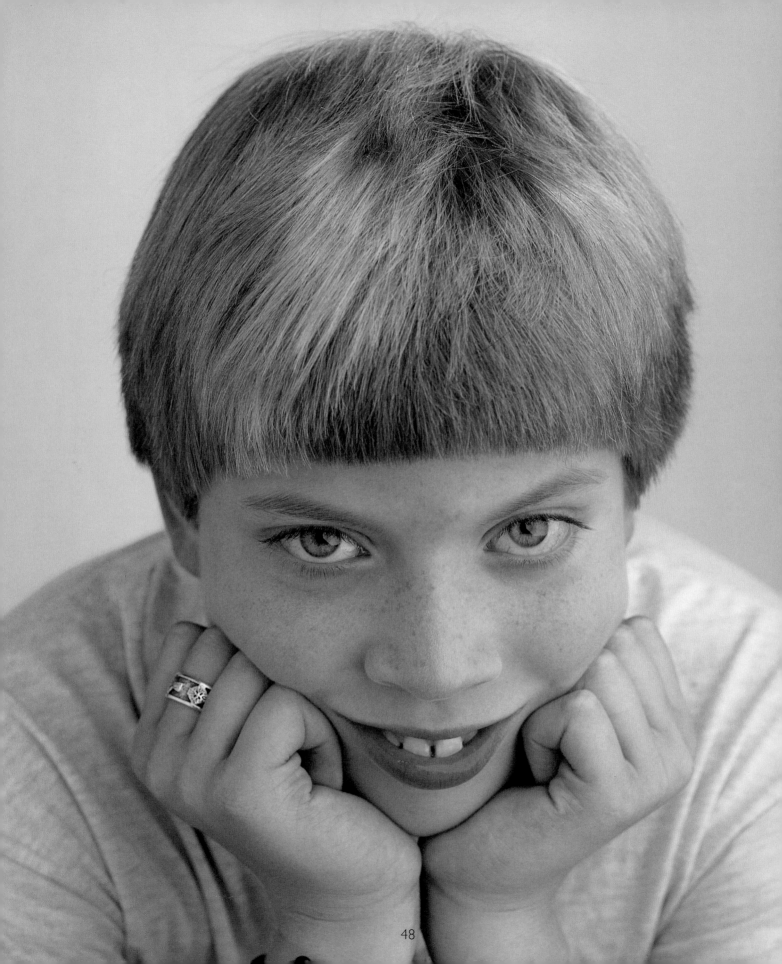

BOYS' ONE-LENGTH SHORT CUT

Hair Type: Medium texture, straight, thick

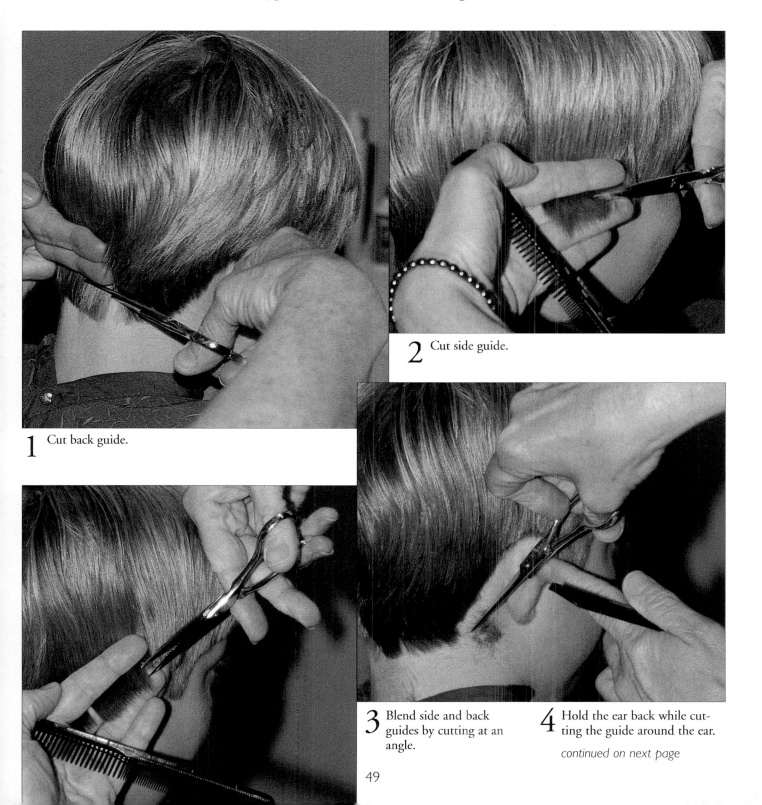

1 Cut back guide.

2 Cut side guide.

3 Blend side and back guides by cutting at an angle.

4 Hold the ear back while cutting the guide around the ear.

continued on next page

49

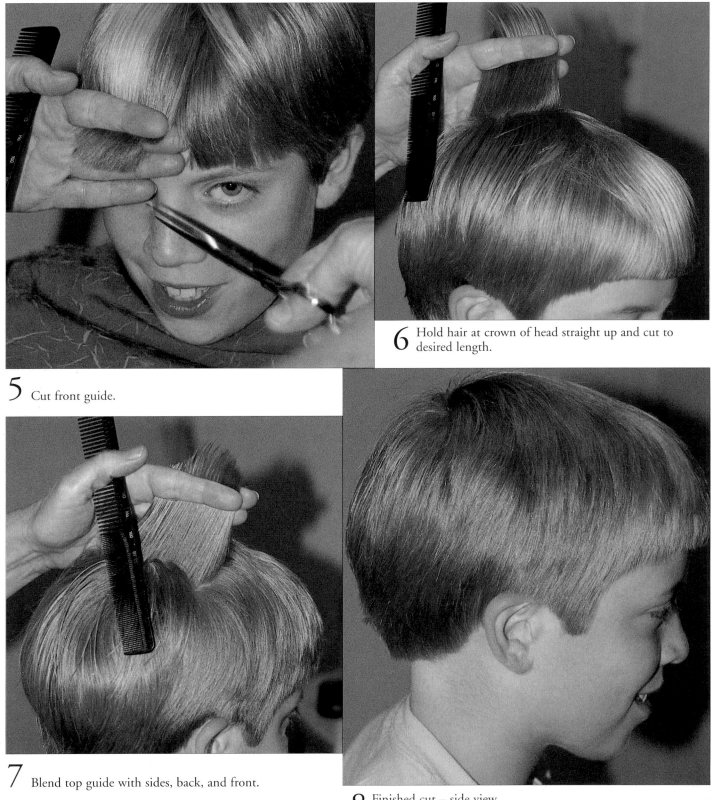

5 Cut front guide.

6 Hold hair at crown of head straight up and cut to desired length.

7 Blend top guide with sides, back, and front.

8 Finished cut – side view.

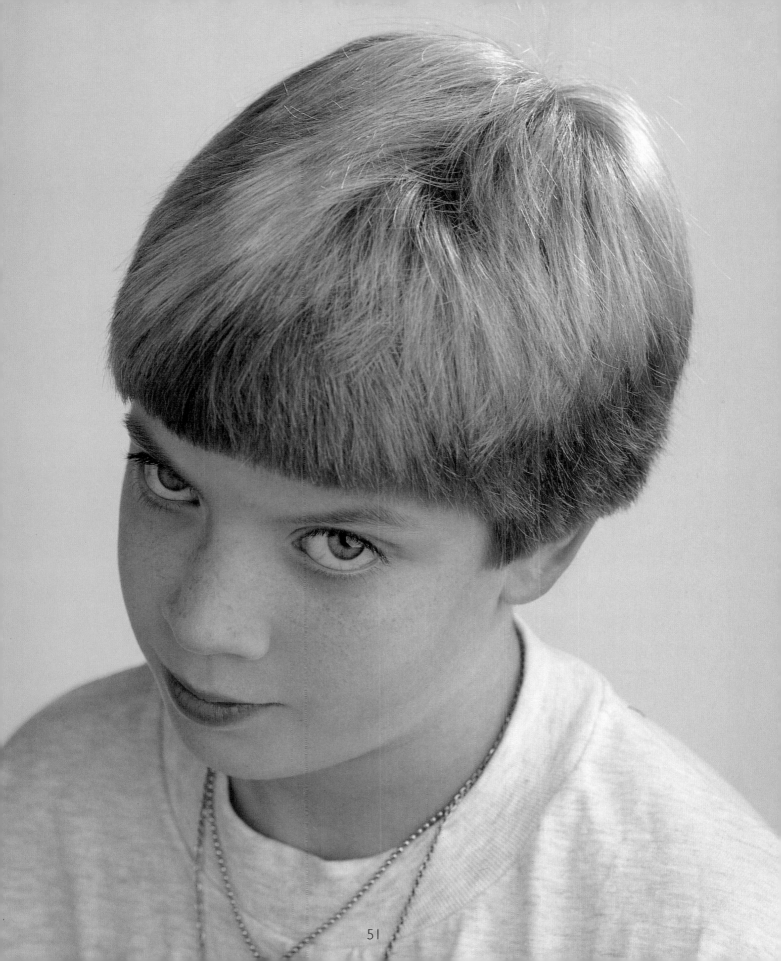

BOYS' SHORT CUT

Hair Type: Fine, wavy

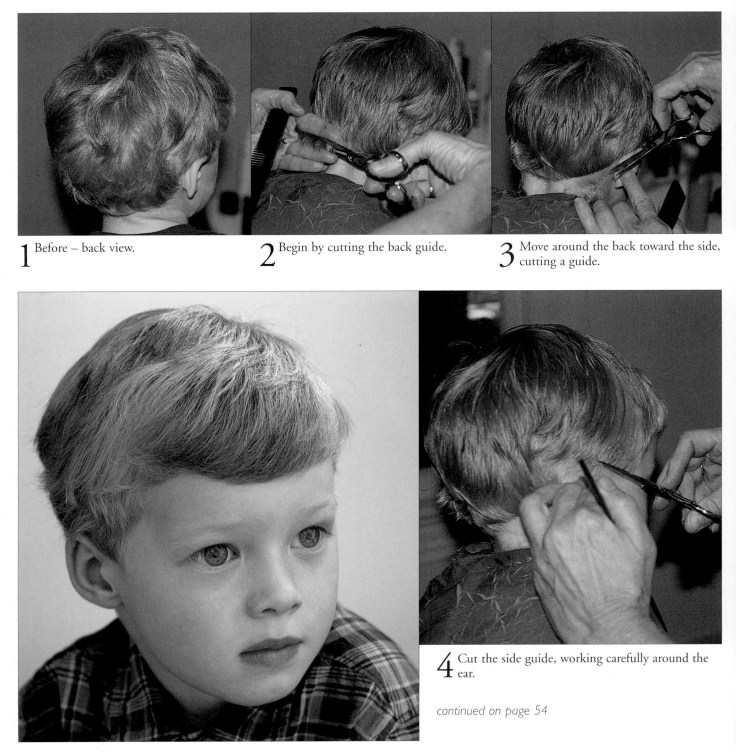

1 Before – back view.

2 Begin by cutting the back guide.

3 Move around the back toward the side, cutting a guide.

4 Cut the side guide, working carefully around the ear.

continued on page 54

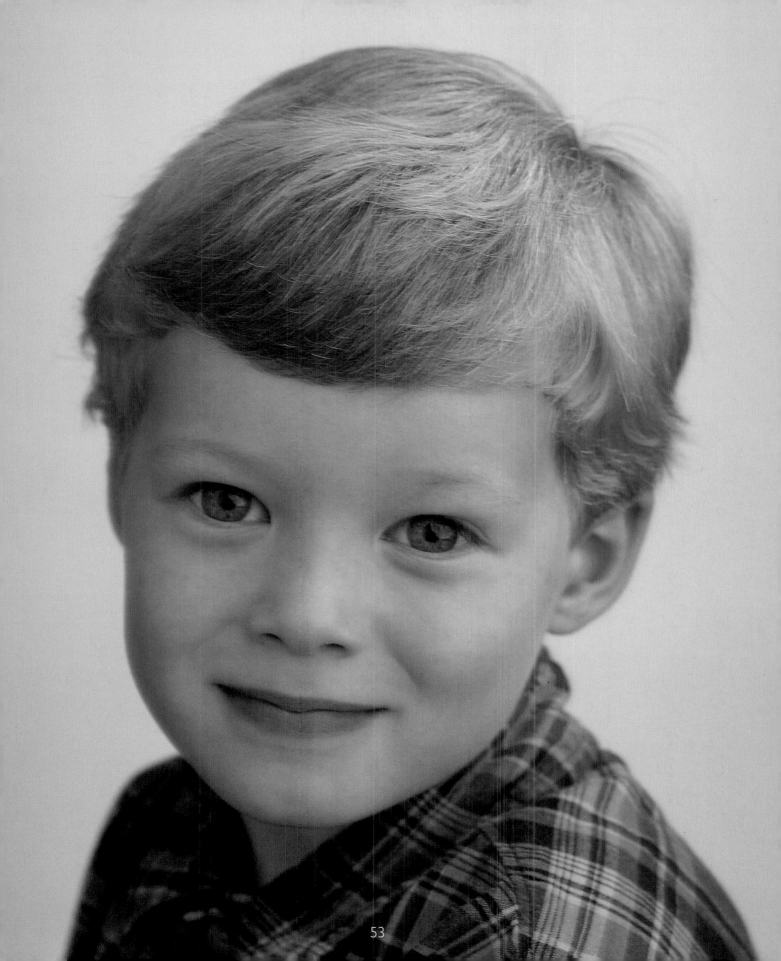

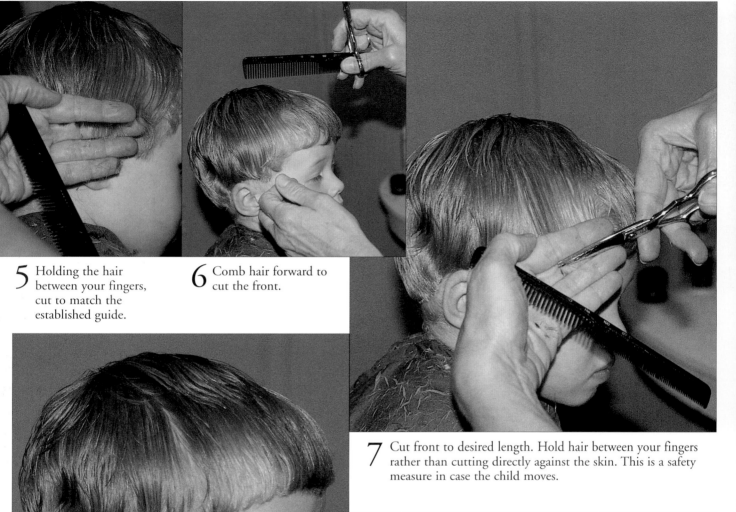

5 Holding the hair between your fingers, cut to match the established guide.

6 Comb hair forward to cut the front.

7 Cut front to desired length. Hold hair between your fingers rather than cutting directly against the skin. This is a safety measure in case the child moves.

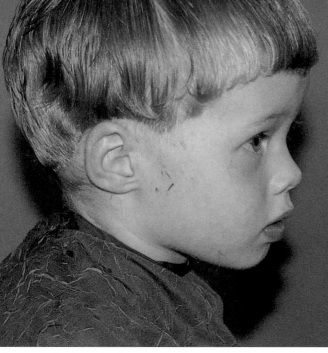

8 Front, back, and side guides are established.

9 Now cut the top guide, holding the hair at the crown of the head straight up.

10 Pick up some of the guide hair with each new section you cut.

11 Blend top and back guides, working one small section (1/4-1/2") at a time. Continue to move around head, following the guide with every section you cut.

12 Clean up the hairline with the clippers.

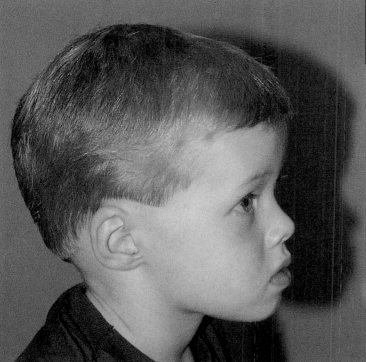

13 The finished cut – side view.

BANGS

Bangs should follow the natural curve of the hairline from temple to temple. Bangs can be wispy or thick, depending on how much hair is cut. Make sure you don't start out with too much hair. It is best to add as you go.
Here's How: Take the hair to be cut and bring it to the nose. Cut the desired amount. This allows the hair to fall naturally with the hair line.

Straight Bangs

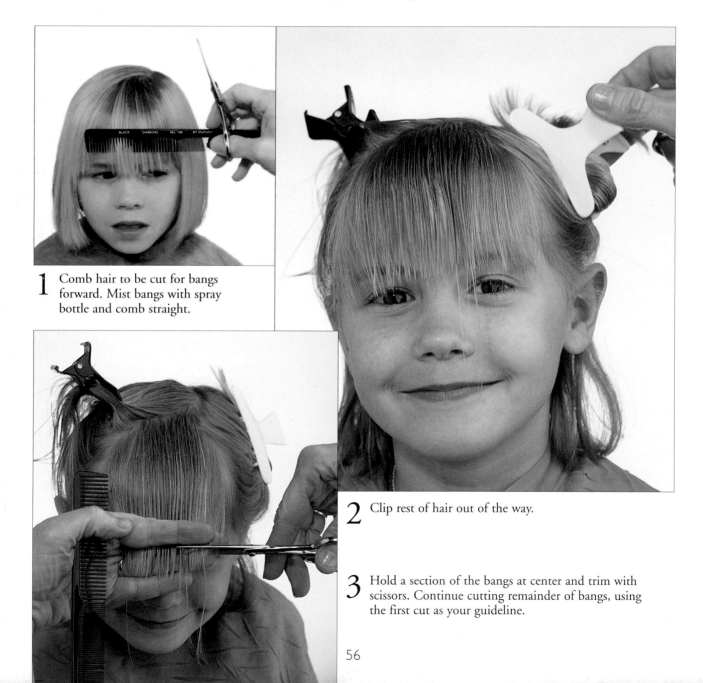

1 Comb hair to be cut for bangs forward. Mist bangs with spray bottle and comb straight.

2 Clip rest of hair out of the way.

3 Hold a section of the bangs at center and trim with scissors. Continue cutting remainder of bangs, using the first cut as your guideline.

56

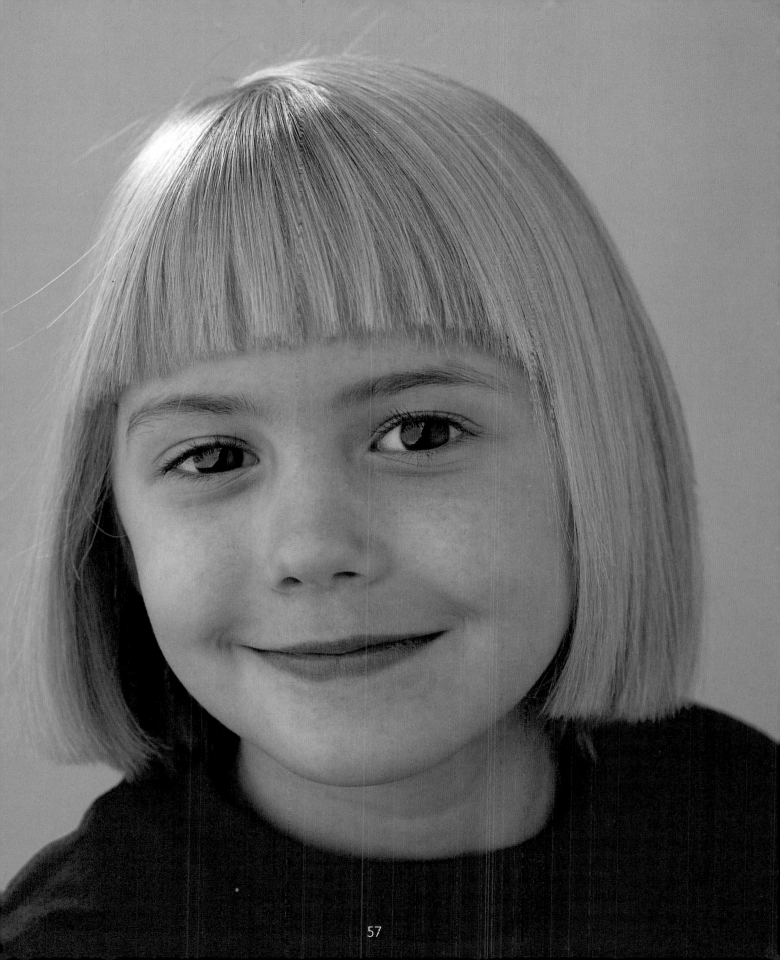

Curved Bangs

Curved bangs are shorter in the center and longer on the sides. To cut them, determine the shortest length (in the center). Cut center section to length desired. Pull all other sections of hair to the center to cut to that same length. (see Fig. 1.) This will result in the edges being slightly longer than the center.

If you want a more drastic difference in the length from center to ends, you will use a different method. First cut the center the length desired, then cut the sides the length desired. Cut hair in between, tapering from the shortest to the longest length on each side. (See Fig. 2)

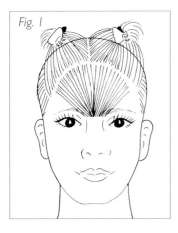

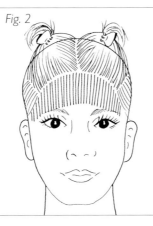

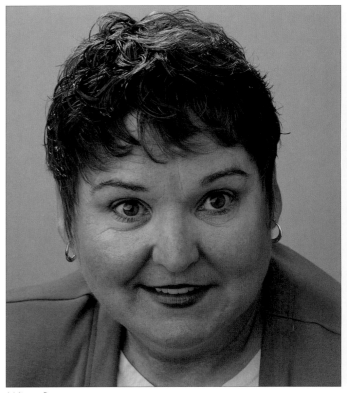

Wispy Bangs

Wispy Bangs

Bangs can be thinned by bringing the hair away from the head at different angles. The more elevation you use, the thinner the bangs will become, creating a wispy look. (See Fig. 3)

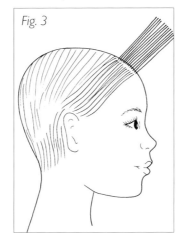

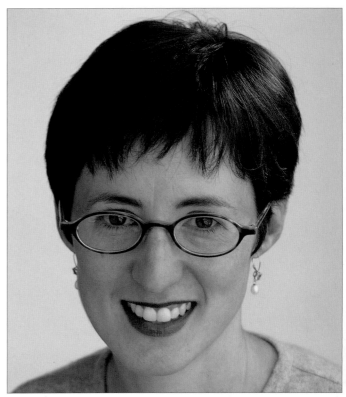

Wispy Bangs

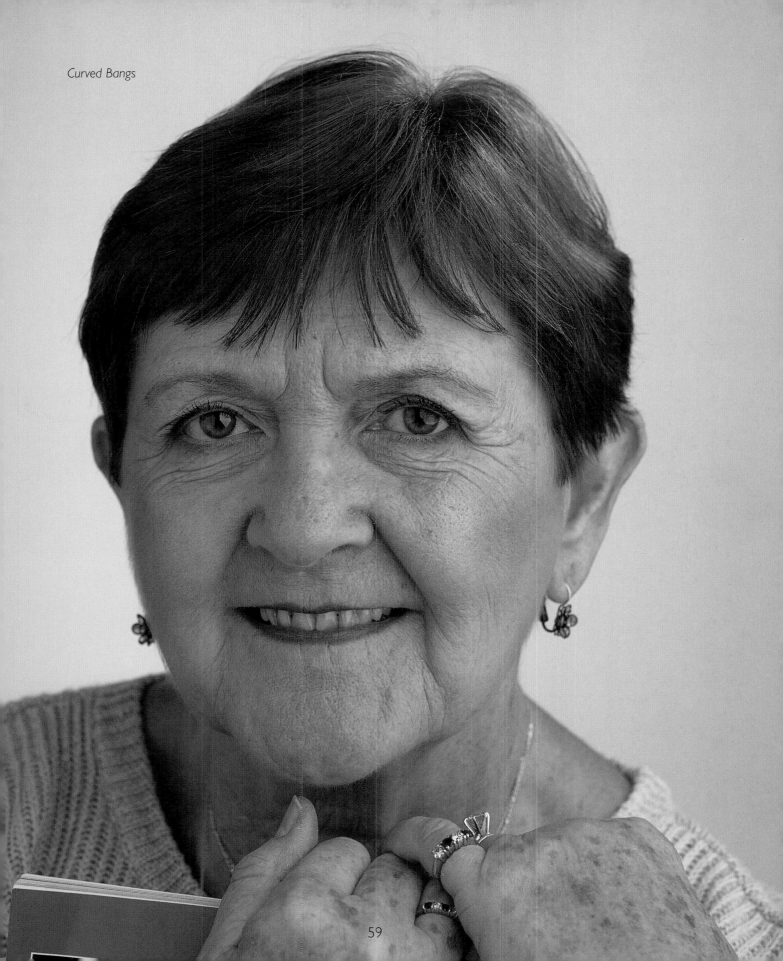

Curved Bangs

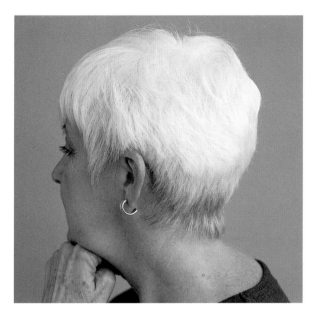

Women's
HAIRCUTTING
Styles

In this chapter I will introduce you to two techniques for cutting women's hairstyles – the one-length cut and the layered cut. Each of these styles can be any length, resulting in a different look. Adding variations like bangs or no bangs will give completely different looks.

The one-length blunt cut is the easiest cut to do. This style looks great on children, on women, and even on some men. This cut can have bangs or not. A short version is perky and easy to care for while the longer version is versatile because it can be worn in a ponytail or braids. The medium version is classic and always "in style."

A layered cut adds another dimension to cutting. (Imagine a cut with a shorter top guide at the crown of the head. By connecting the top guide and bottom guide, a layered cut is created.) The lengths of the top and bottom guides determine the lengths of the layers.

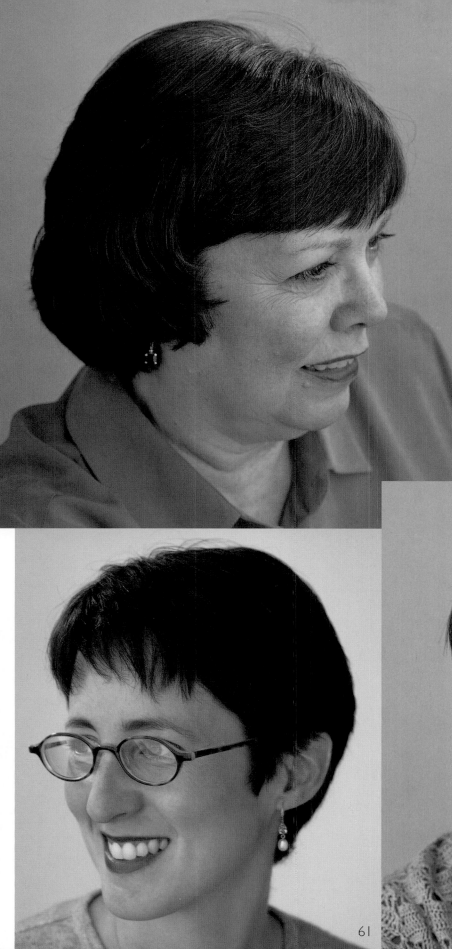

Pictured at left:

Short
One-Length Cut

See pages 65-69 for step-by-step instructions.

Pictured below:

Short
Layered Cuts

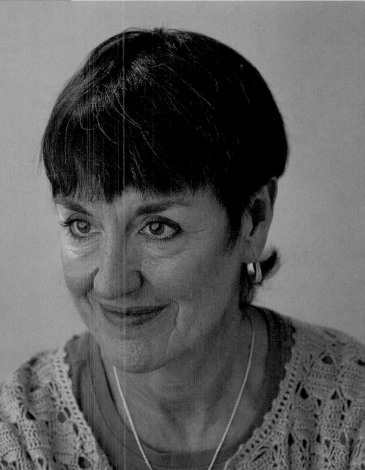

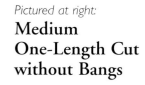

Pictured at left:

**Medium
One-Length Cut
with Bangs**

See pages 70-73
for step-by-step
instructions.

Pictured at right:

**Medium
One-Length Cut
without Bangs**

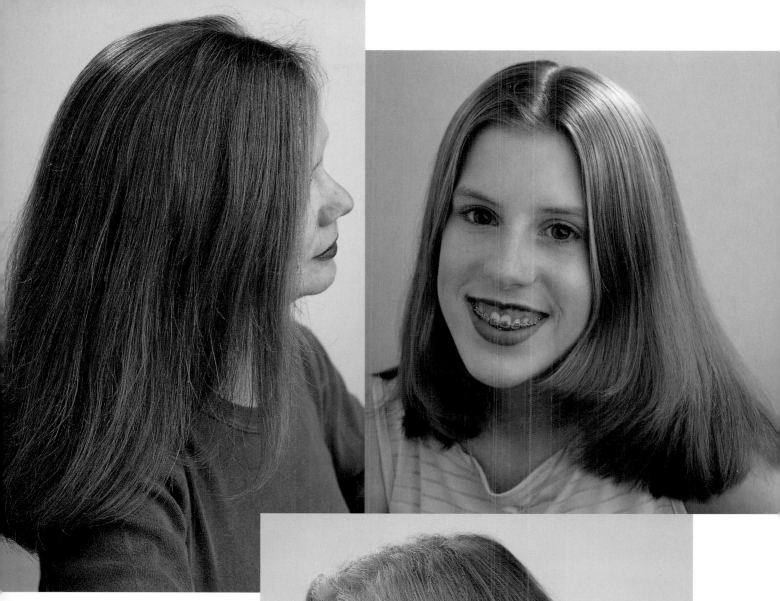

Pictured above and at right:

**Long
One-Length Cuts**

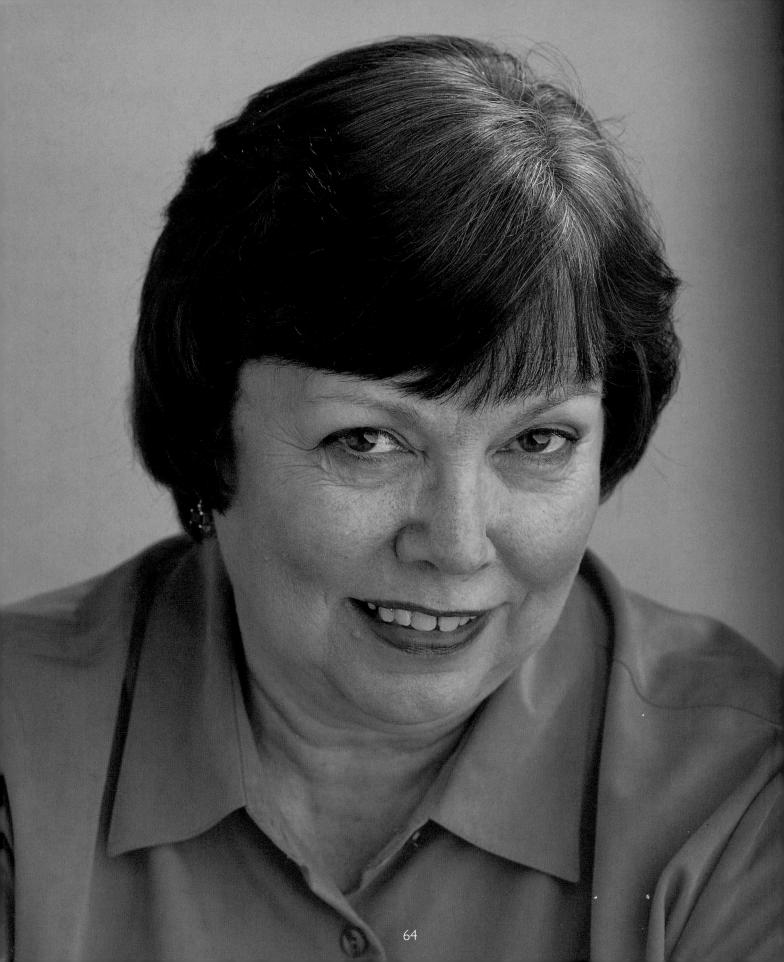

SHORT ONE-LENGTH CUT WITH BANGS

For this cut, all the hair is cut one-length, forming a straight blunt edge. This cut is the easiest to create. This blunt cut was done on thick wavy hair and bangs were added. Because the hair is wavy it doesn't have the straight-across, even look that straighter, thinner hair would have.

Hair Type Shown: Thick, wavy, medium texture

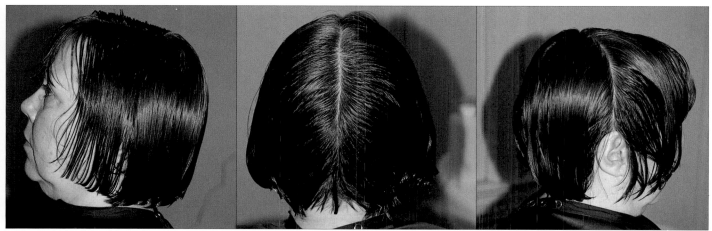

1 Hair is wet and ready to cut. Comb all hair down straight and smooth.

2 Begin sectioning hair. Part hair from center of forehead to center of nape of neck.

3 Continue sectioning hair. Part hair from ear to ear.

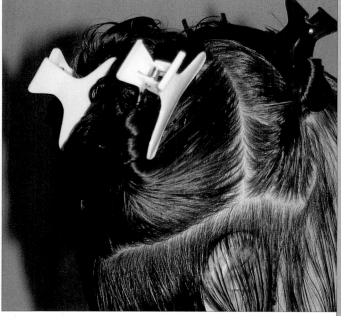

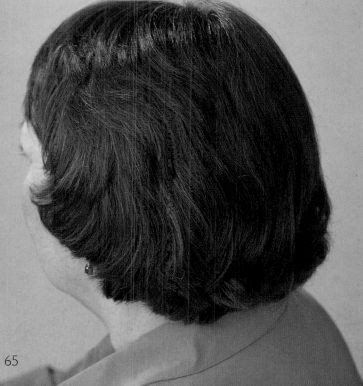

4 Secure each section with a butterfly clip, leaving a 1" section around the perimeter of the head. This will be the guide.

continued on next page   *Finished back view*

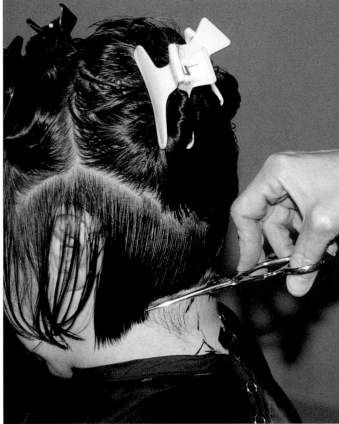

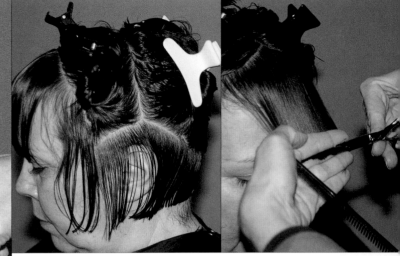

6 The side hair will be cut the same length as the back. In this photo, the side hair has not yet been cut.

7 Cut the front guide.

5 Cut the back guide to the desired length. This back length is cut just at the hairline.

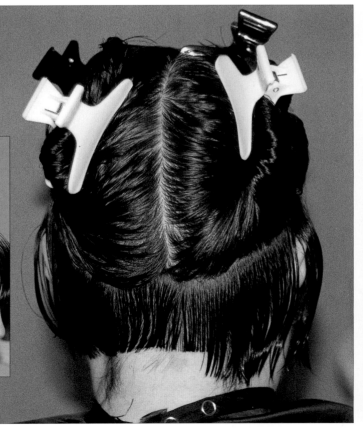

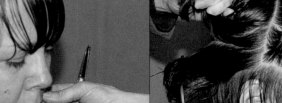

8 Check the front and side guides for desired length and accuracy. Pull strands forward to see if they are the same lengths. Adjust if necessary.

9 After the guides are cut, begin pulling the hair out of the butterfly clips, working one 1" section at a time. The remaining sections of hair will be cut to the guides.

10 Notice the difference in length. This 1" section will be cut to the same length as the guide.

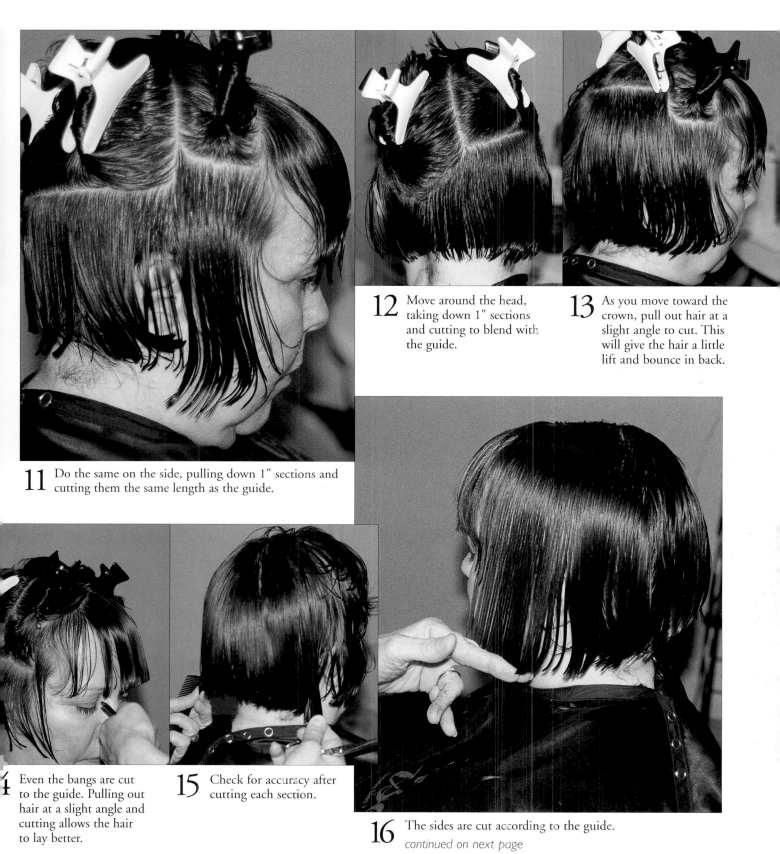

11 Do the same on the side, pulling down 1" sections and cutting them the same length as the guide.

12 Move around the head, taking down 1" sections and cutting to blend with the guide.

13 As you move toward the crown, pull out hair at a slight angle to cut. This will give the hair a little lift and bounce in back.

14 Even the bangs are cut to the guide. Pulling out hair at a slight angle and cutting allows the hair to lay better.

15 Check for accuracy after cutting each section.

16 The sides are cut according to the guide.
continued on next page

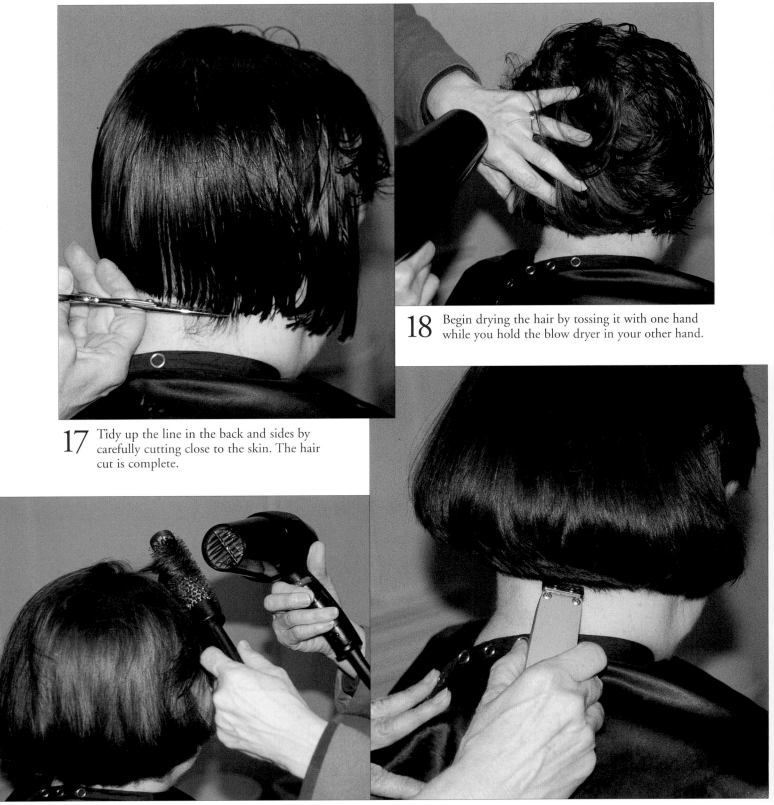

17 Tidy up the line in the back and sides by carefully cutting close to the skin. The hair cut is complete.

18 Begin drying the hair by tossing it with one hand while you hold the blow dryer in your other hand.

19 **Optional:** To help ends turn under, use a round hair brush. Use your wrist to twist the brush.

20 **Optional:** Clean hair from the neck with clippers.

Fig. 1. Cut the back guides. All hair will be cut to the length of the guides.

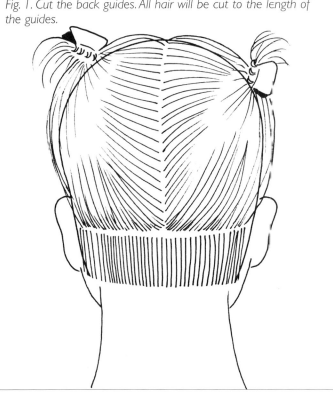

Fig. 2. As you let down the sections, continue to cut and match the guides.

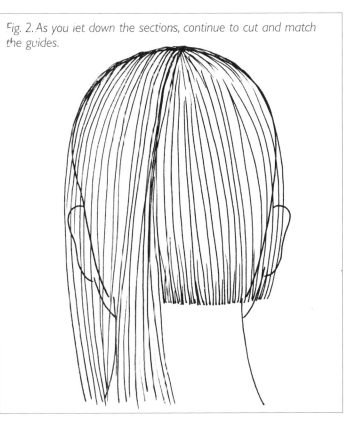

Fig. 3. Cut the back guides to the length desired.

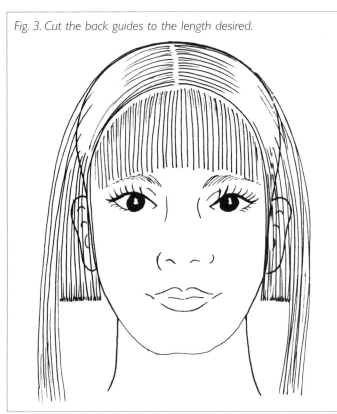

Fig. 4. Continue cutting around the perimeter of hair, cutting the side guides to desired length.

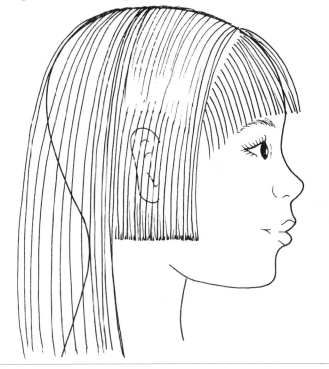

MEDIUM ONE-LENGTH CUT WITH BANGS

This is a good cut for thin very straight hair because it gives the hair more volume and is a natural cut for straight hair.

Hair Type Shown: Straight, thin, fine texture

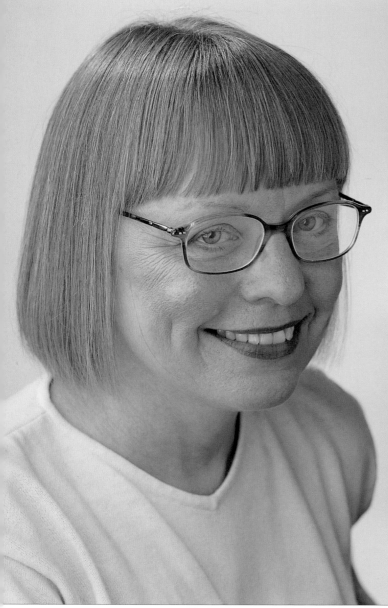

Finished cut

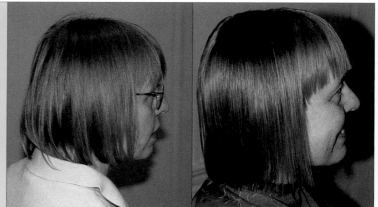

1 Before. Hair grows at different lengths, so when the hair hasn't been trimmed it tends to get uneven edges and look "scraggly."

2 Hair is washed, combed, and ready to cut.

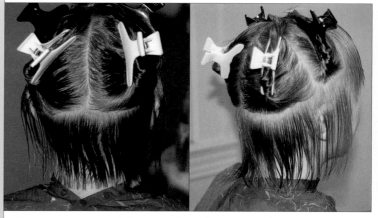

3 Hair is sectioned for ease of cutting. Hair is parted from forehead to nape and ear to ear and clipped.

4 Leave a 1" section around the perimeter. This section of hair will be cut to the desired length and all other hair will be cut to match this guide.

continued on page 72

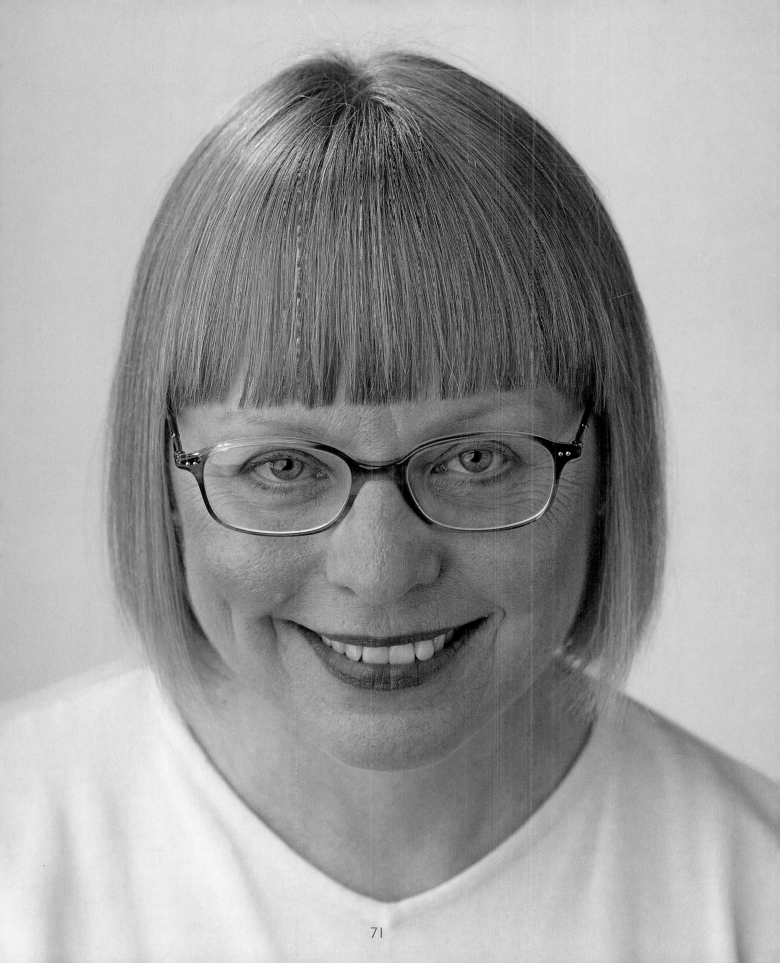

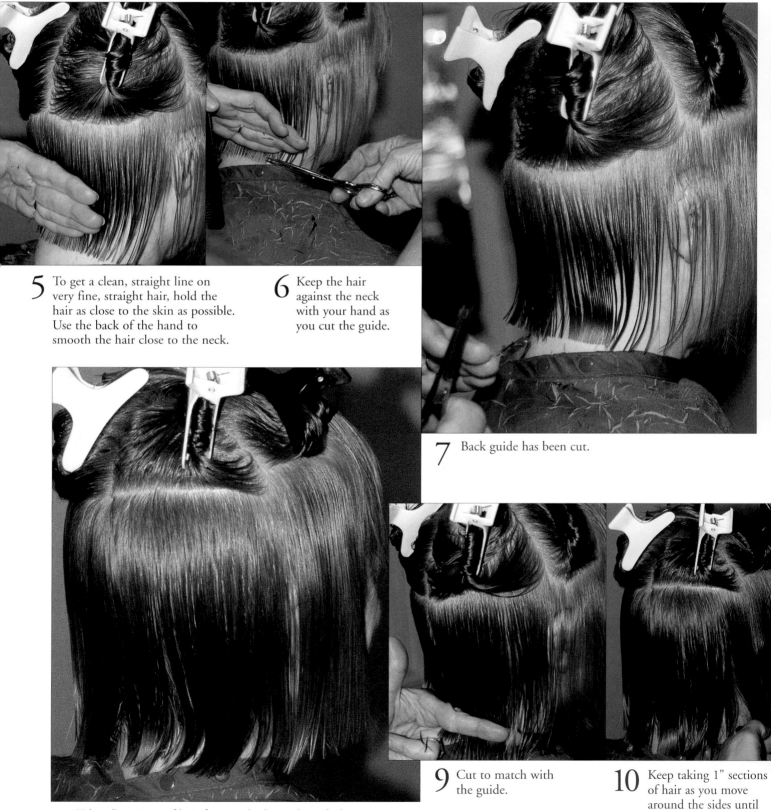

5 To get a clean, straight line on very fine, straight hair, hold the hair as close to the skin as possible. Use the back of the hand to smooth the hair close to the neck.

6 Keep the hair against the neck with your hand as you cut the guide.

7 Back guide has been cut.

8 Take 1" sections of hair from each clip and comb down.

9 Cut to match with the guide.

10 Keep taking 1" sections of hair as you move around the sides until all hair is cut.

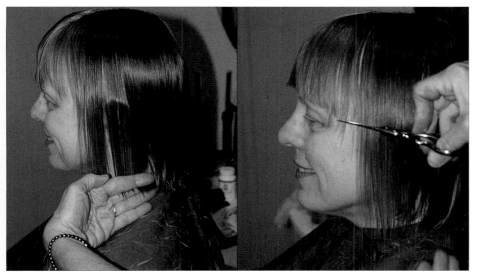

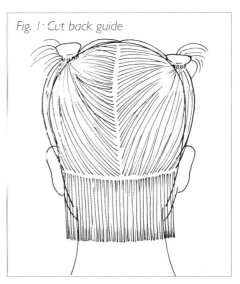

Fig. 1: Cut back guide

11 As you cut new sections, compare them to the guide to keep even.

12 Finish the cut by trimming the bangs.

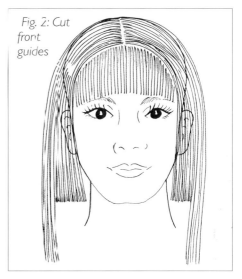

Fig. 2: Cut front guides

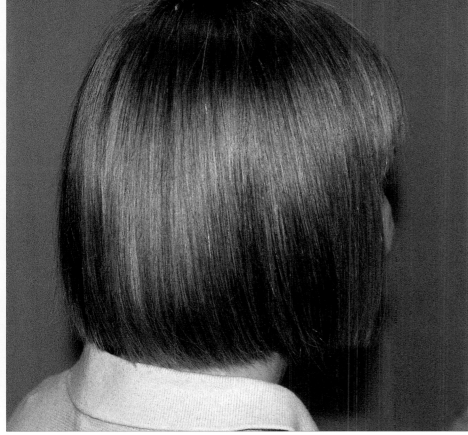

13 As you cut new sections, compare them to the guide to keep even.

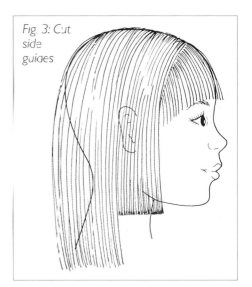

Fig. 3: Cut side guides

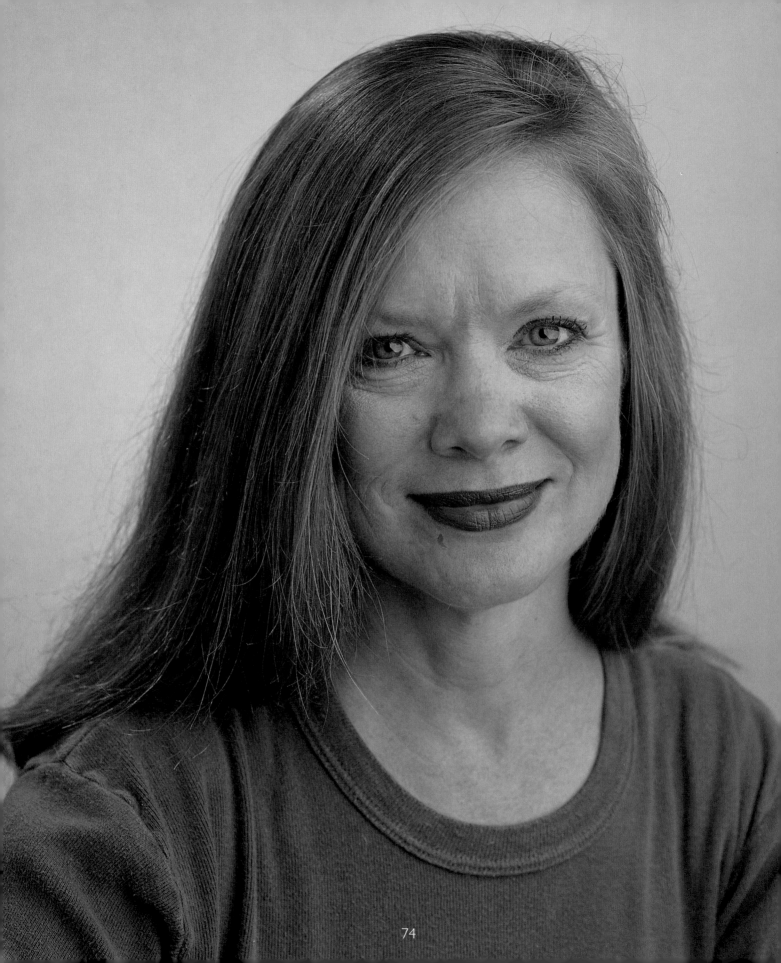

LONG ONE-LENGTH CUT

Hair Type: Wavy, thin, fine texture

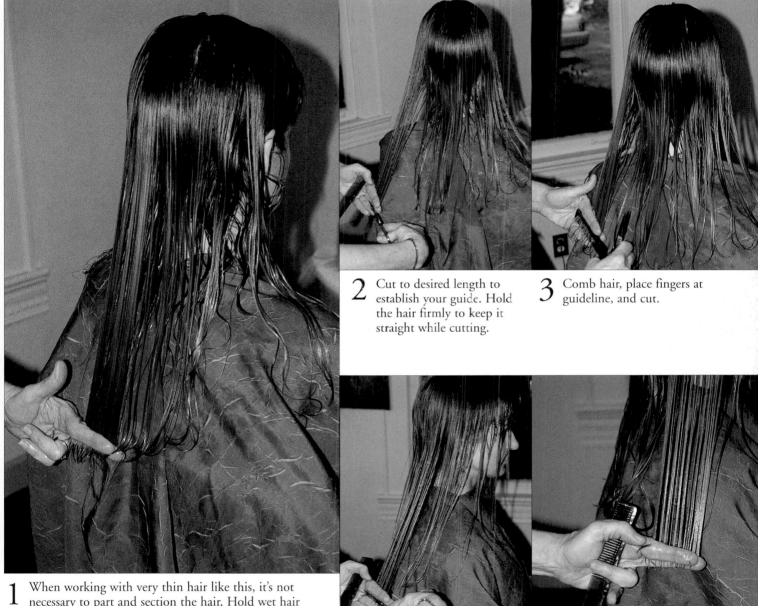

1 When working with very thin hair like this, it's not necessary to part and section the hair. Hold wet hair between your fingers to determine the amount to be removed.

2 Cut to desired length to establish your guide. Hold the hair firmly to keep it straight while cutting.

3 Comb hair, place fingers at guideline, and cut.

4 Following the guide, cut to length.

5 Comb the hair straight down and hold the hair firmly as you cut.

continued on page 77

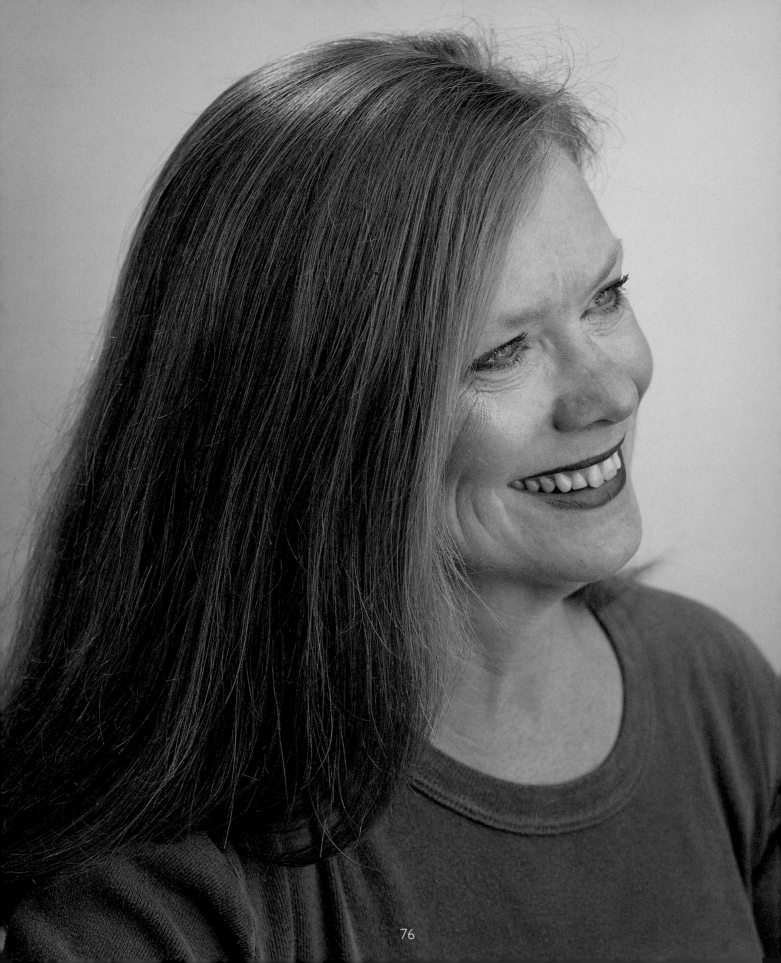

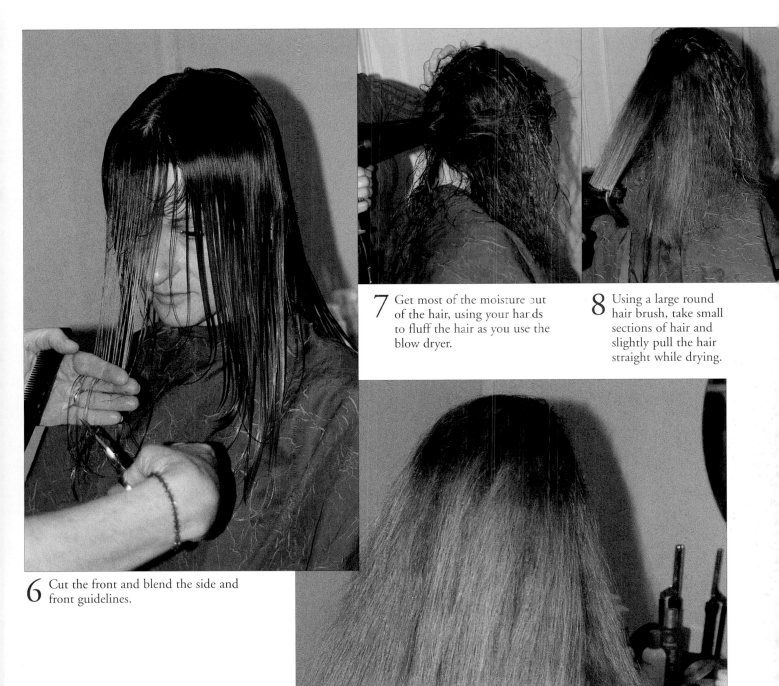

6 Cut the front and blend the side and front guidelines.

7 Get most of the moisture out of the hair, using your hands to fluff the hair as you use the blow dryer.

8 Using a large round hair brush, take small sections of hair and slightly pull the hair straight while drying.

9

The finished cut – back view.

OTHER LONG ONE-LENGTH CUTS

This one-length cut was done on thin, fine, curly hair. Because it is curly it will curl-up at ends and give soft, less blunt edge. The sides were cut slightly shorter at an angle to frame the face.

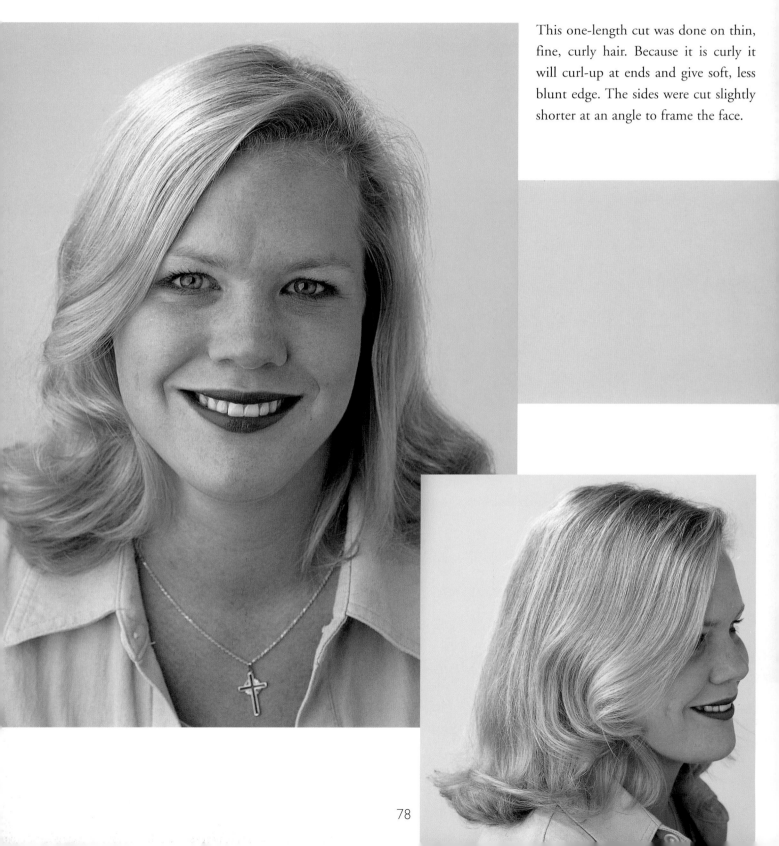

This one length cut was done on dense (thick) hair with a fine texture. The front guide was cut just slightly shorter and angled to frame the face nicely.

SHORT LAYERED CUT

Hair Type: Fine, slightly wavy

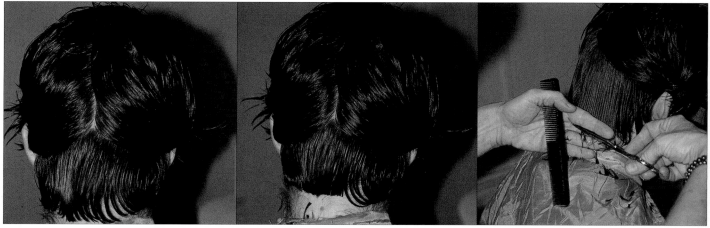

1 Section hair from crown to center of nape of neck, leaving 1". When hair is very short, it is hard to hold in a butterfly clip. In this case the hair is pulled aside and pinned in place.

2 Cut hair in back to length desired. This is the guide.

3 Comb hair down over guide. Hold the hair slightly away from the head and cut along the guideline.

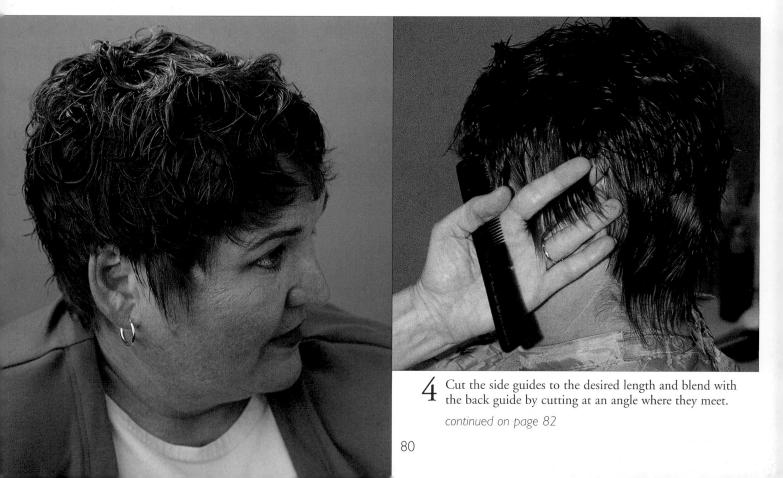

4 Cut the side guides to the desired length and blend with the back guide by cutting at an angle where they meet.

continued on page 82

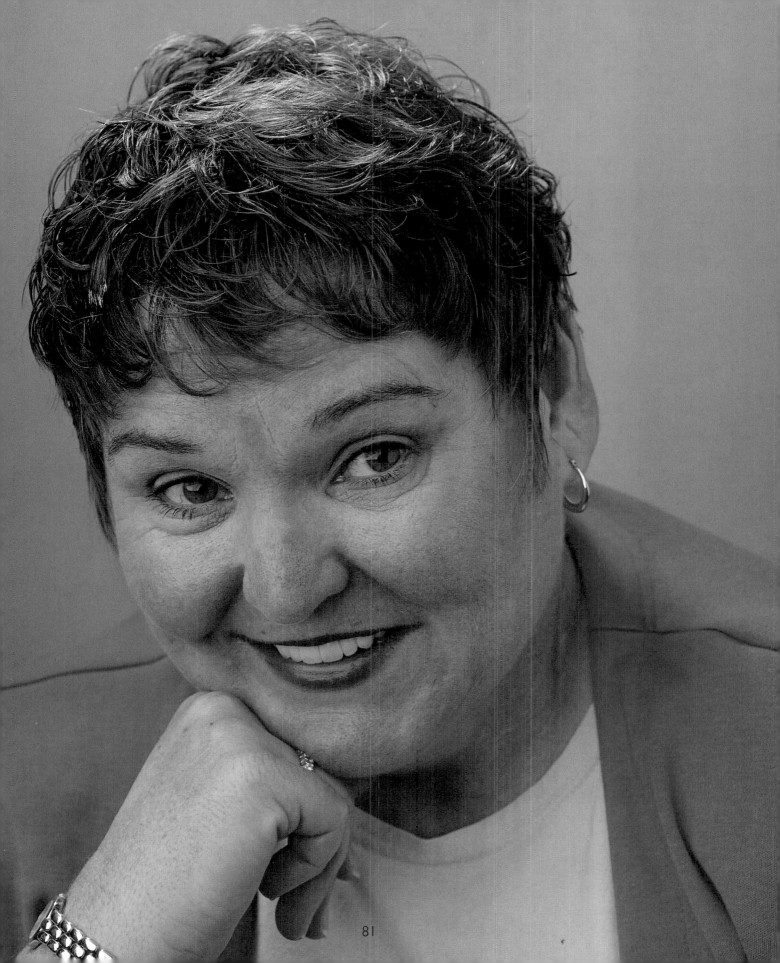

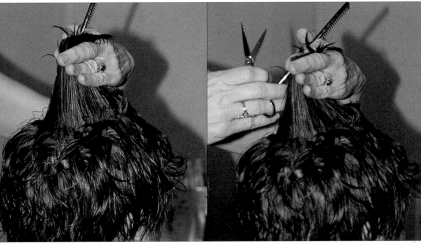

5 To cut top, hold the hair straight up (180 degree angle) from the crown and determine length.

6 Cut the top guide.

7 To layer the remainder of hair, work your way down the back, pulling hair out from the scalp at a 90-degree angle and cutting to the length of the guides. Blend the top guide and the back guide.

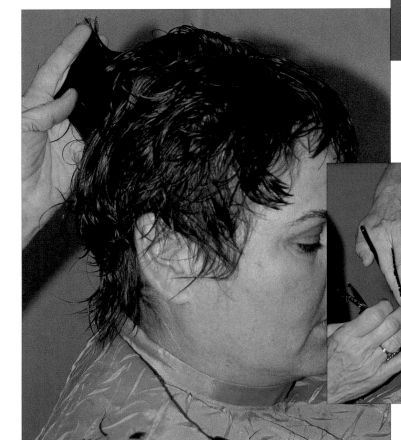

8 This shows the hair that was pulled out, cut to the proper length. The cut is made on the far side of the fingers that hold the hair out.

9 Continue to work down the back of the head, cutting hair to proper length, following length determined by guides.

10 Now work from the crown to the front.

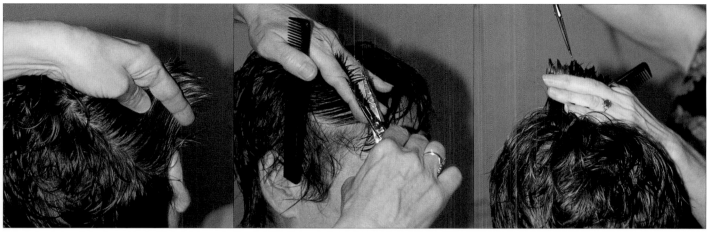

11 Pull sections from the sides, pulling out at the 90-degree angle. Cut to blend. Blend the sides behind the ears with the back.

12 Blend the sides with the top.

13 To create a feathered look, hold sections of the hair up and cut directly into the hair, creating v-shaped cuts. Do this all over the head.

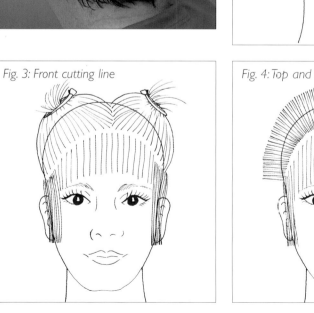

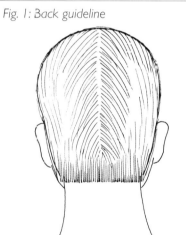

Fig. 1: Back guideline

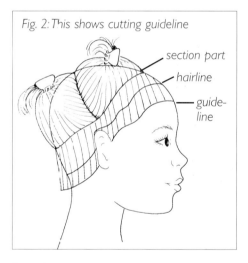

Fig. 2: This shows cutting guideline

section part

hairline

guide-line

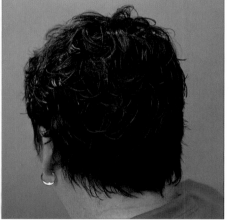

Fig. 3: Front cutting line

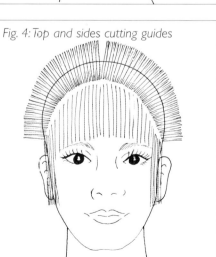

Fig. 4: Top and sides cutting guides

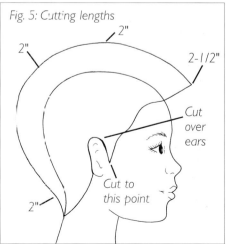

Fig. 5: Cutting lengths

2"

2"

2-1/2"

Cut over ears

Cut to this point

2"

OTHER SHORT LAYERED CUTS

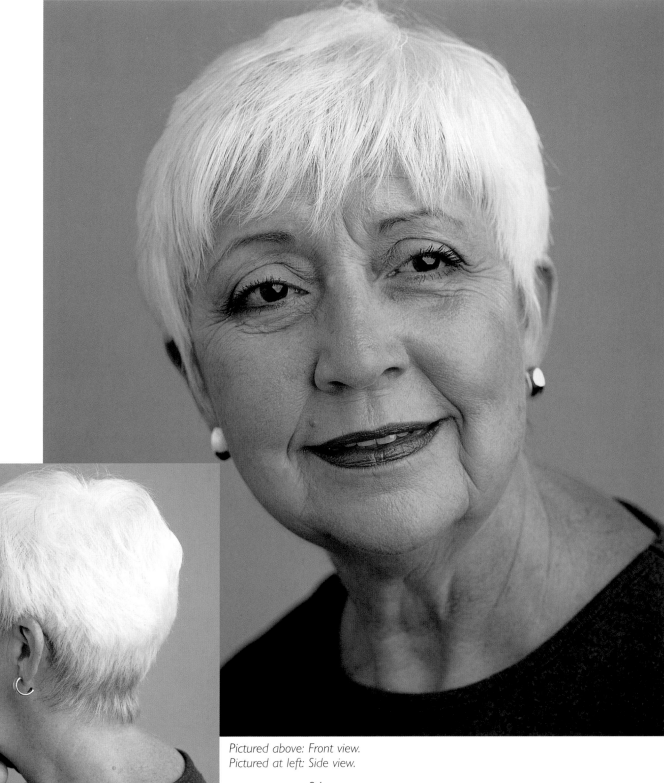

Pictured above: Front view.
Pictured at left: Side view.

84

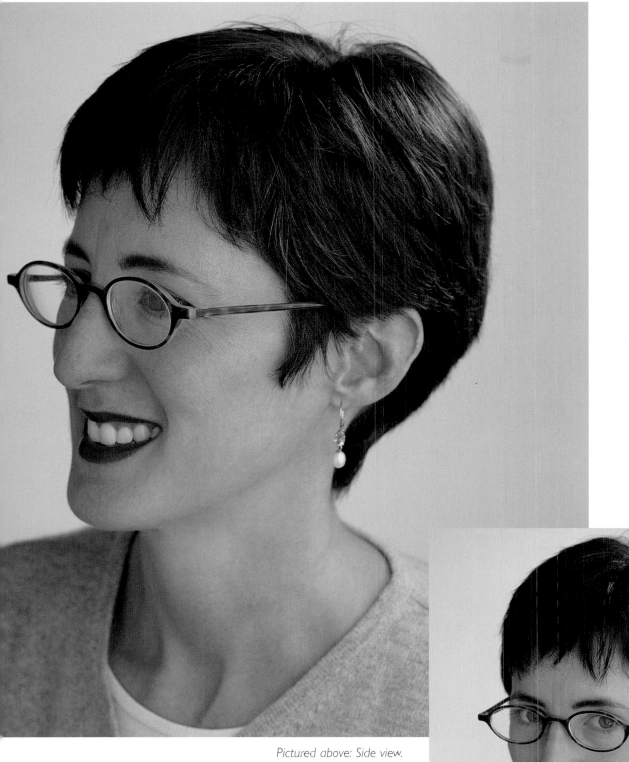

Pictured above: Side view.
Pictured at right: Front view.

SHORT LAYERED WISPY CUT

Hair Type: Wavy, medium texture, medium thick

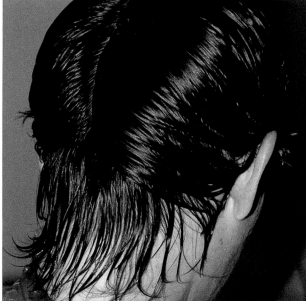

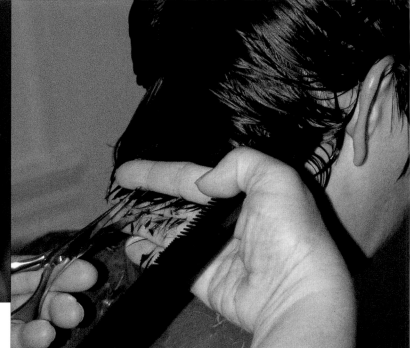

1   Wet hair, combed and ready to cut. Part and section hair. Clip if necessary.

2   To cut guide, begin at the back. Hold the hair out from the head and cut into the hair at an angle rather than straight across. This will feather the layers.

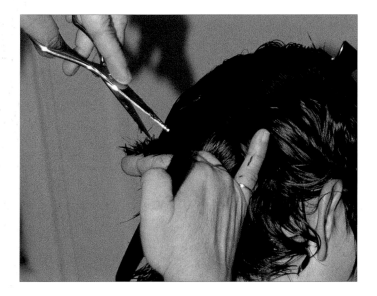

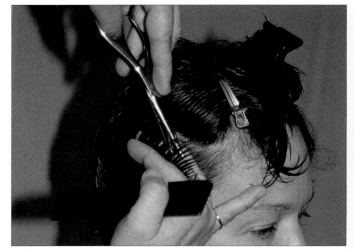

3   Take 1" sections of hair and move diagonally on the head from back to front. Lift each 1" section straight out (90-degree angle) from the head to cut into the ends, in a "v" rather than cutting straight across.

4   Continue to cut, lifting each section and moving up the back and around to the sides. As you cut, blend each section with the bottom guide.

continued on page 89

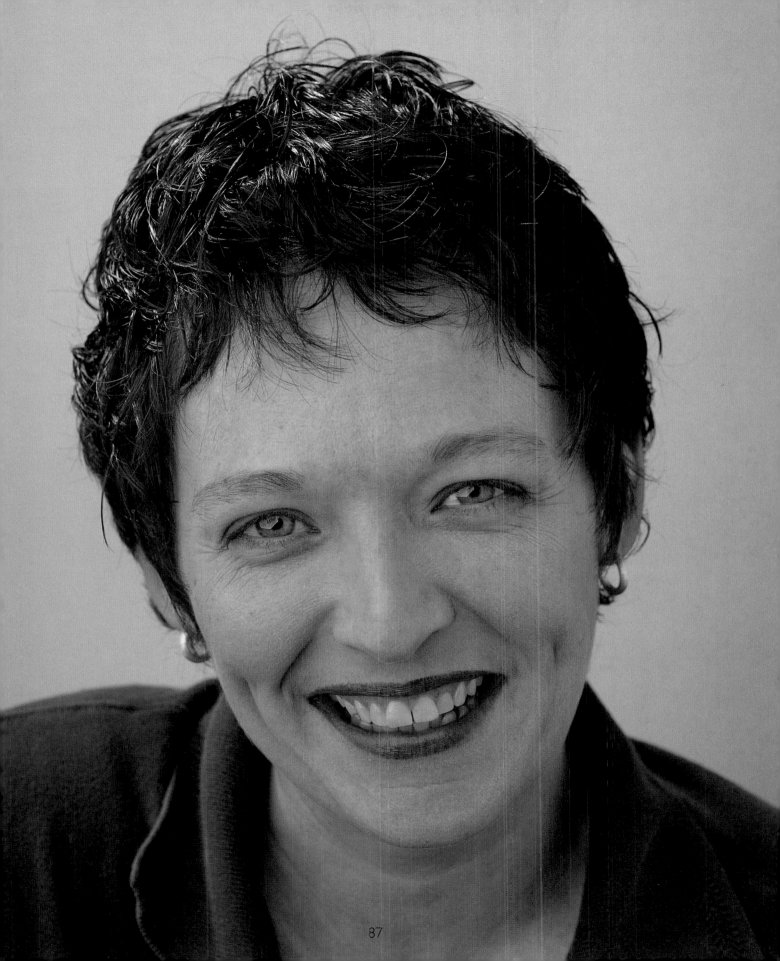

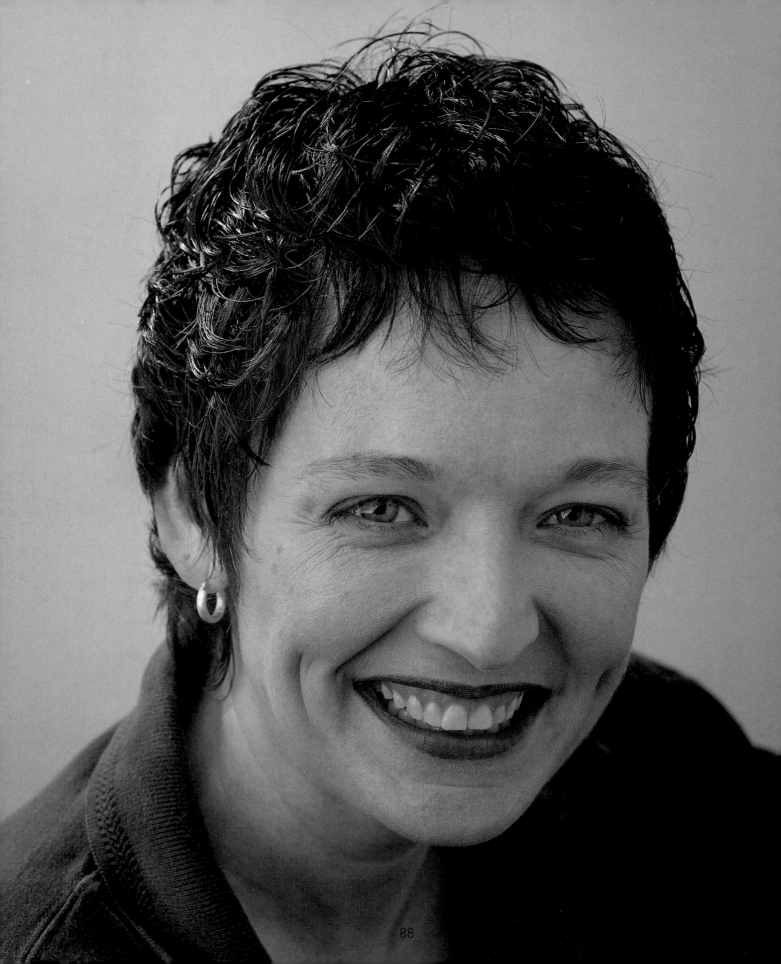

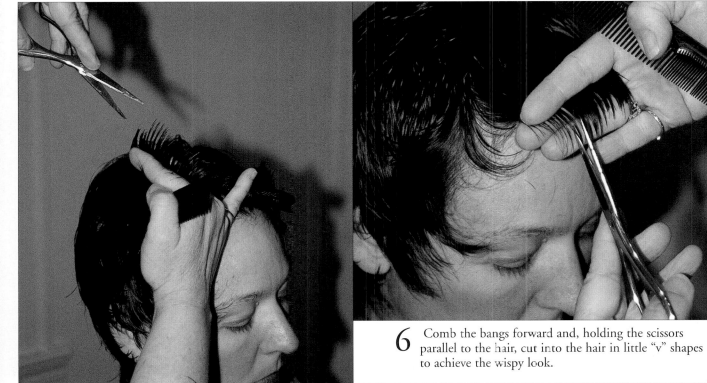

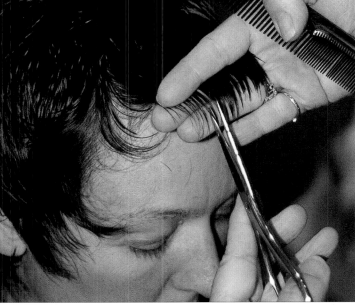

6 Comb the bangs forward and, holding the scissors parallel to the hair, cut into the hair in little "v" shapes to achieve the wispy look.

5 Take 1" sections from the clip at the top of the head and cut to blend with the sides and back.

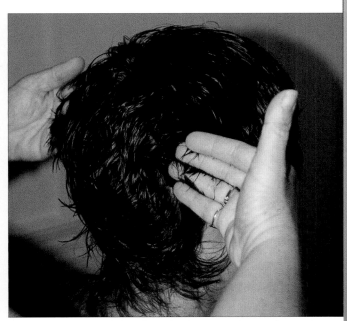

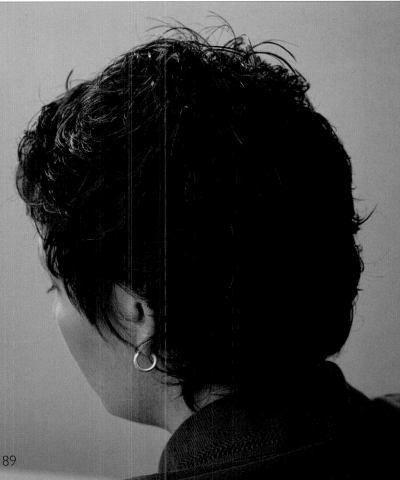

7 Check the cut by pulling the hair straight out from the head with your fingers, feeling and observing to be sure it is even.

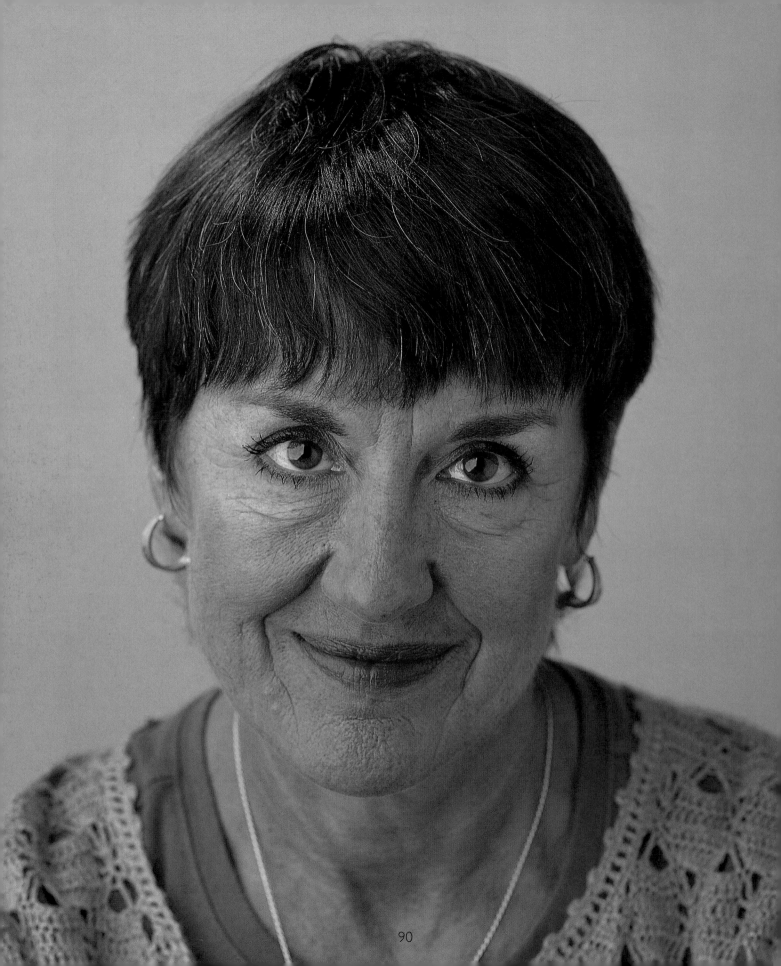

SHORT ONE-LENGTH CUT WITH LAYERED BACK

Hair Type: Fine, straight, somewhat thin

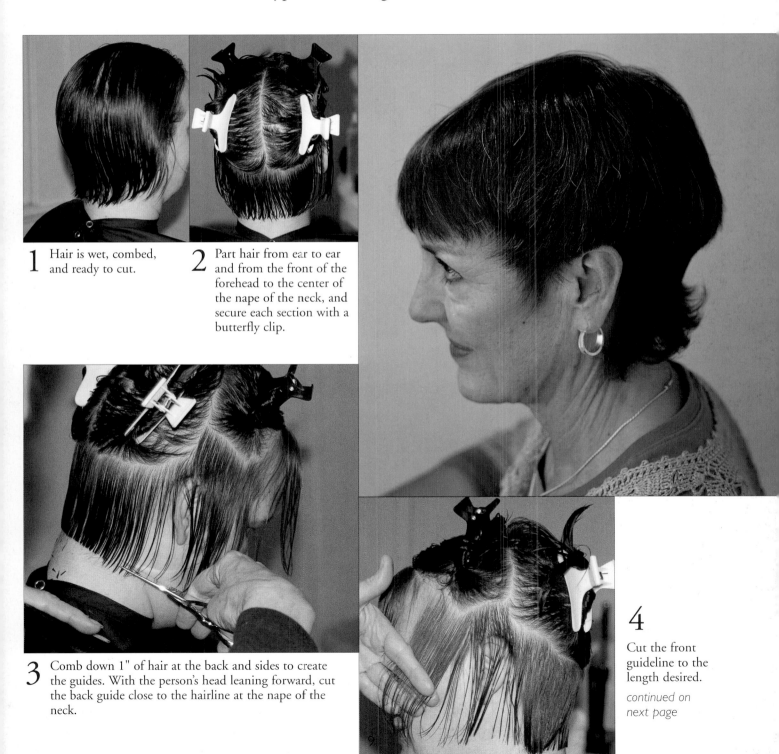

1 Hair is wet, combed, and ready to cut.

2 Part hair from ear to ear and from the front of the forehead to the center of the nape of the neck, and secure each section with a butterfly clip.

3 Comb down 1" of hair at the back and sides to create the guides. With the person's head leaning forward, cut the back guide close to the hairline at the nape of the neck.

4 Cut the front guideline to the length desired.

continued on next page

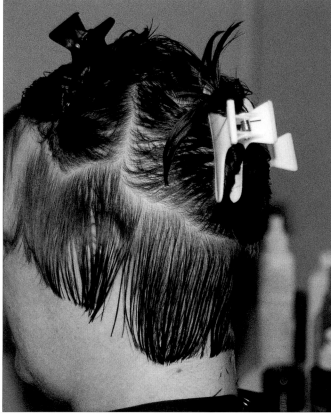

5 Back and front guides and bangs have been cut.

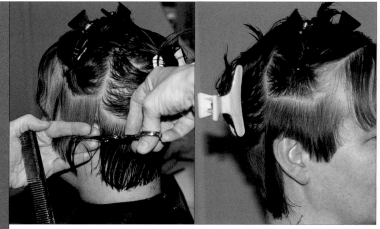

6 For a sculptured look, cut the hair on the sides above the ears, following the shape of the ears.

7 Back, front and side guides have been cut.

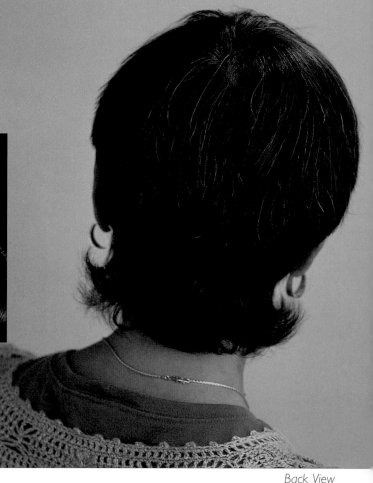

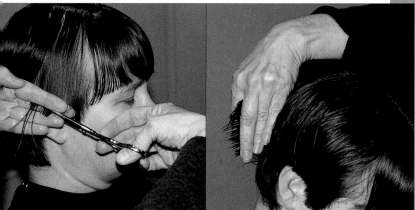

8 To continue, comb all side sections down over the guides. Cut each section even with the guides.

9 To layer the back, hold sections of hair straight out from the head at a 90-degree angle. Cut even with back guide. Cut all back sections, working one section at a time and blending the sections as you go.

Back View

OTHER SHORT LAYERED CUTS

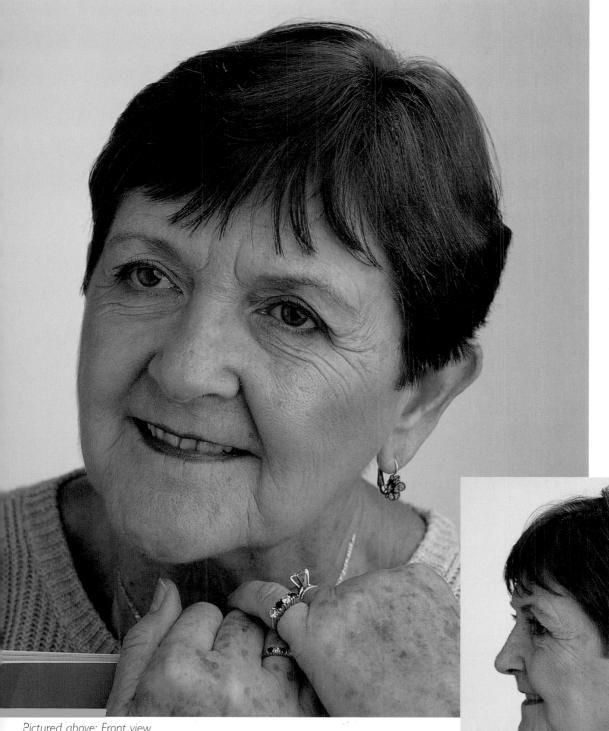

Pictured above: Front view.

Pictured at right: Side view.

MEDIUM LAYERED CUT

This style has very subtle layers. This is created by pulling the hair out from the head at smaller angles.

Hair Type: Straight, thick, medium texture

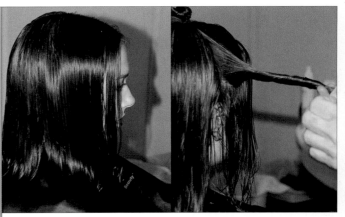

1 Before. Hair is wet, combed smooth, and ready to cut.

2 Section hair. Part hair from ear to ear and from center front to center back. Because the hair is long, I twisted the sections (twisting makes it easier to clip up longer hair) and secured with butterfly clips.

3 Hair is parted and clipped. A 1" section is left at the back for cutting the guide.

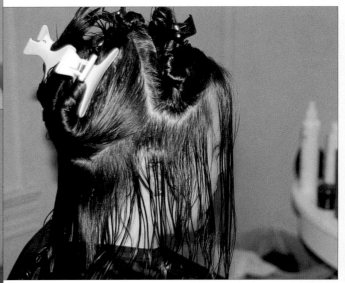

4 A 1" section of hair also is combed down on the sides and front for the guide.

continued on page 96

94

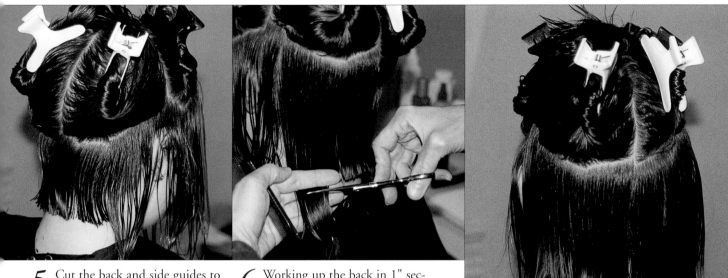

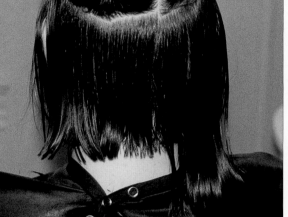

5 Cut the back and side guides to the desired length.

6 Working up the back in 1" sections, take hair from the clips and cut to the guide.

7 Continue across the back, cutting each section even with the guide.

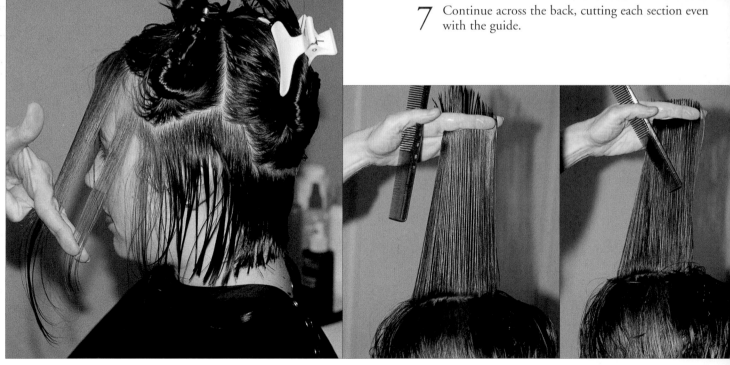

8 Move to the front and cut even with the side the guides, angling hair down slightly toward the face.

9 The shortest layer in this cut is on top. After you've determined how short the shortest layer will be, hold a section of hair from the crown straight up at a 180-degree angle. This will be the top guide.

10 Cut the top guide, holding the hair straight up. This photo shows the top guide cut. The hair is cut on the far side of the fingers, using them as a guide to cut a straight line.

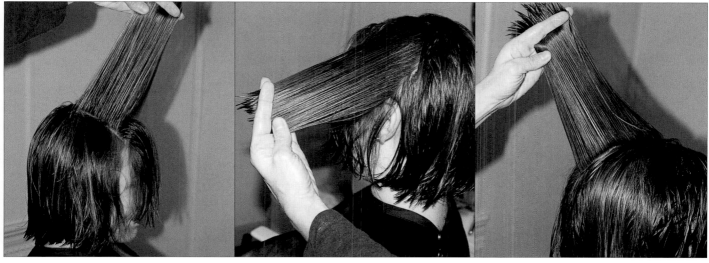

11 The top and front is cut one 1" section at time, blending each section with the top guide. Continue to cut the entire top.

12 Cut the sides by holding them out at a 45-degree angle, cutting them even with the guide. Blend the side guide to the top guide.

13 Blend the top guide to the back guide.

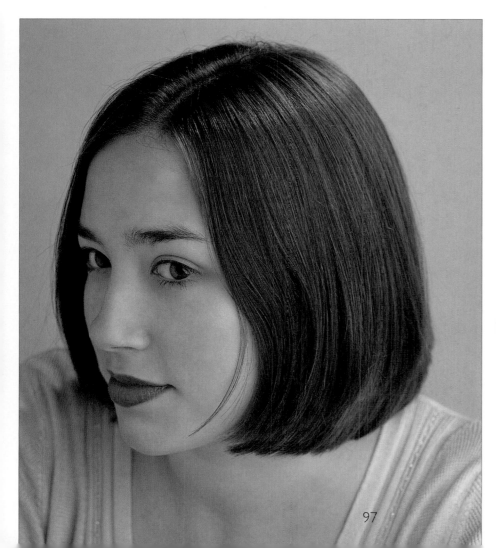

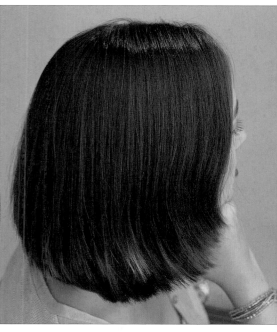

Pictured above: Back view.

Pictured at left: Side view.

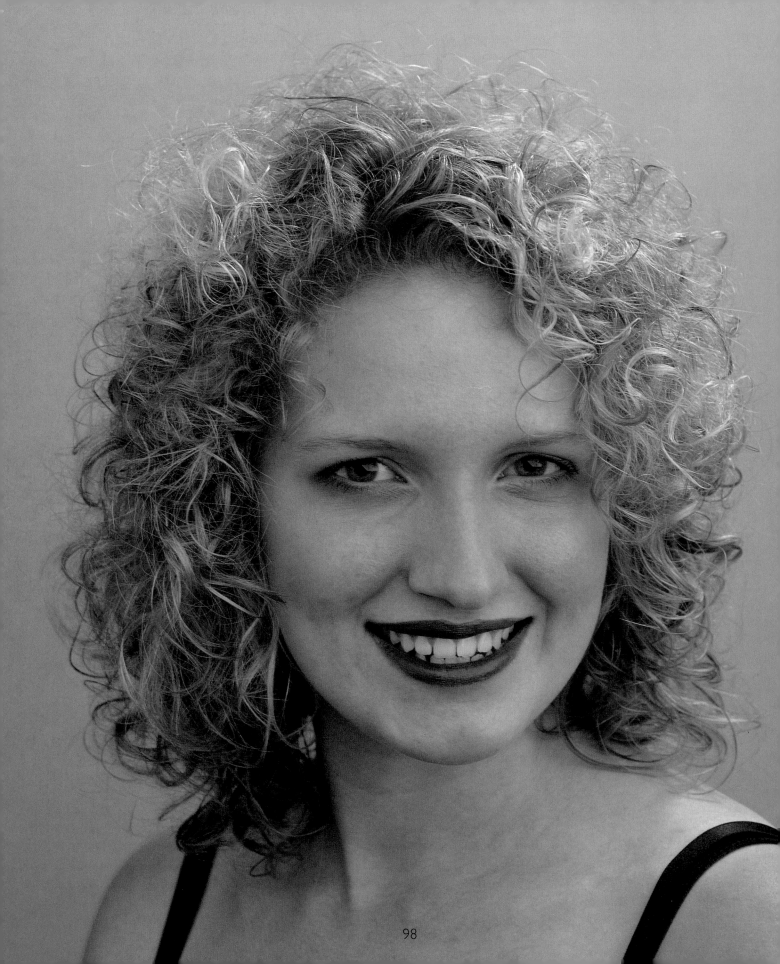

LONG LAYERED CUT

This cut is a modified bob cut. The shortest layer is the top. So all hair sections are pulled up to meet the top for the cutting length.

Hair Type: Curly, thick, medium texture

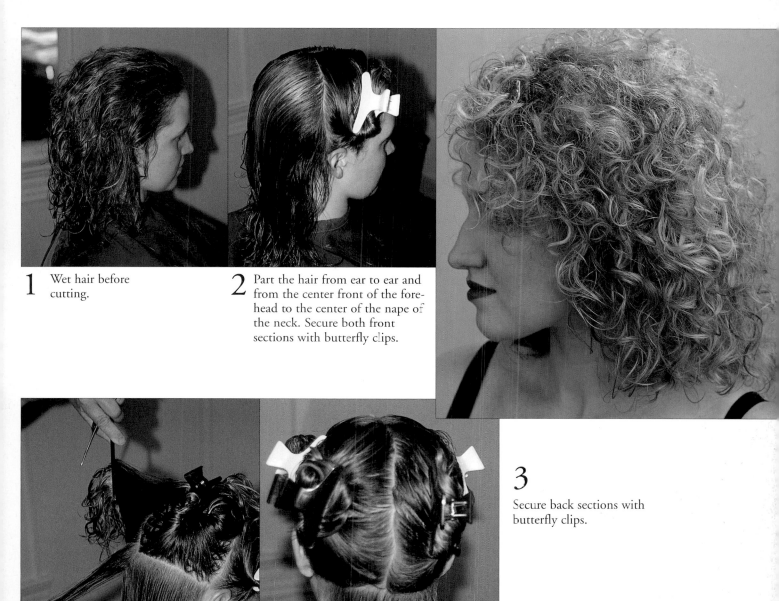

1 Wet hair before cutting.

2 Part the hair from ear to ear and from the center front of the forehead to the center of the nape of the neck. Secure both front sections with butterfly clips.

3 Secure back sections with butterfly clips.

4 Leave a 1" section of hair at the back to establish a guideline.

continued on page 101

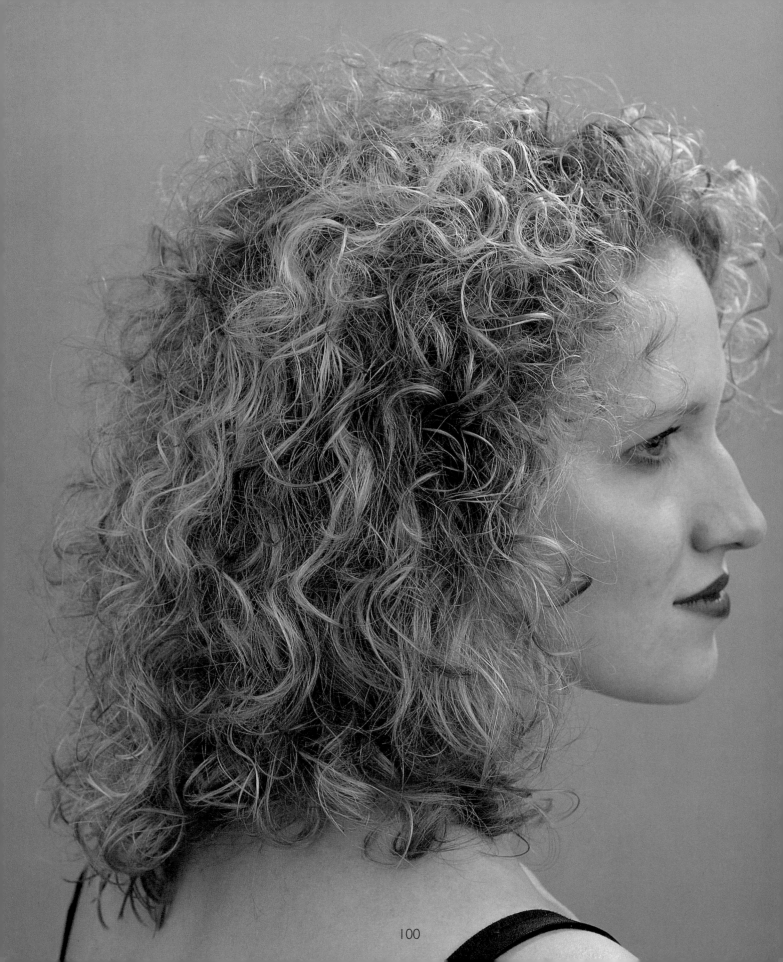

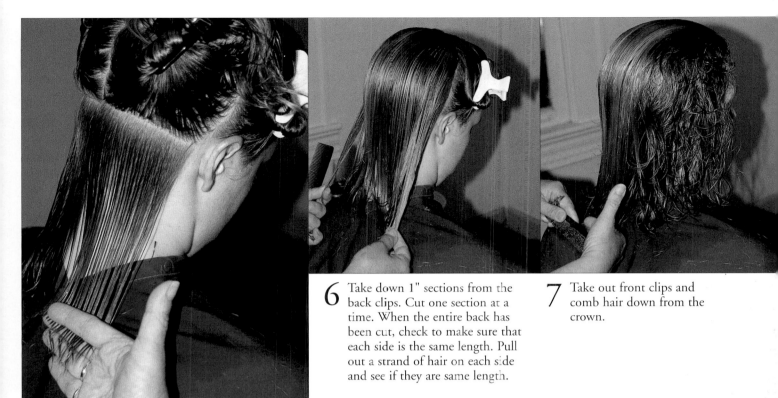

6 Take down 1" sections from the back clips. Cut one section at a time. When the entire back has been cut, check to make sure that each side is the same length. Pull out a strand of hair on each side and see if they are same length.

7 Take out front clips and comb hair down from the crown.

5 Cut the guideline to the desired length, checking to be sure it is even.

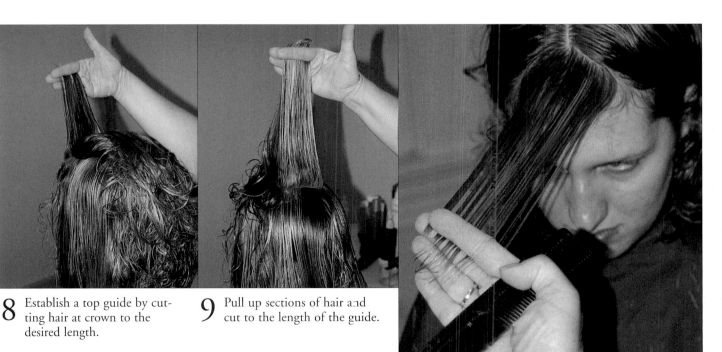

8 Establish a top guide by cutting hair at crown to the desired length.

9 Pull up sections of hair and cut to the length of the guide.

10 Cut the front guide to the desired length.

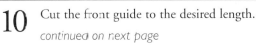

continued on next page

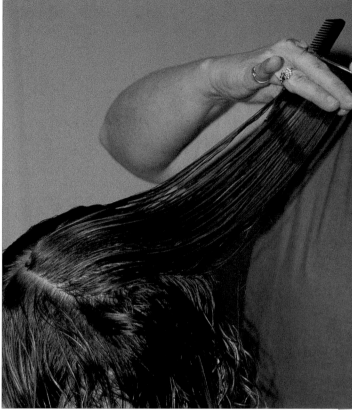

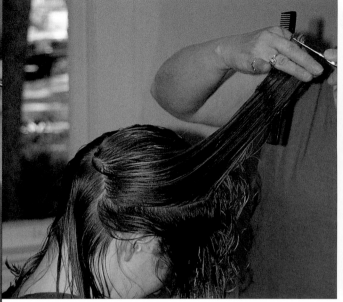

12 Pick up 1" sections of hair from the sides and cut to blend with the top guide.

11 Blend the top guide to the front guide.

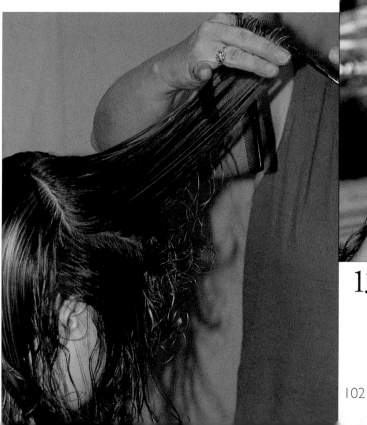

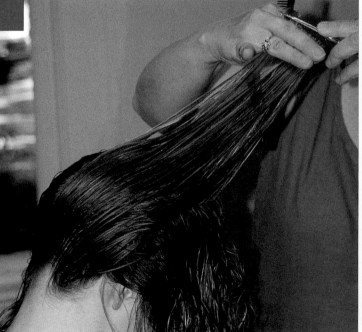

13 Move toward the back, pulling out hair at a 90-degree angle and cutting the hair to blend the back hair with the sides.

14 Join the back hair to the top and cut.

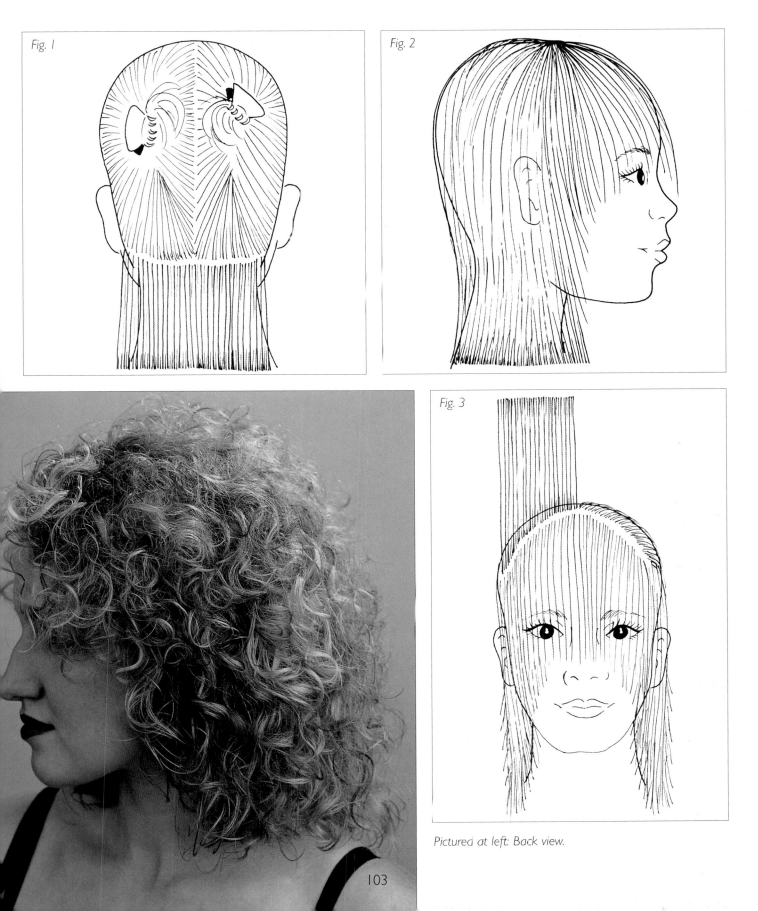

Fig. 1

Fig. 2

Fig. 3

Pictured at left: Back view.

103

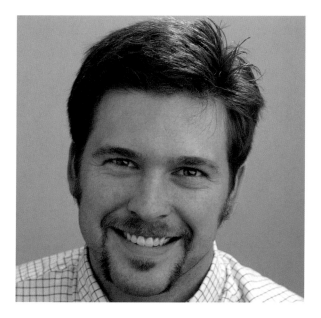

Men's
HAIRCUTTING
Styles

This section shows basic short styles for men. The techniques can also be used for women, boys, and girls who want short hair. Men's (or anyone's) hair may be too short to be held in butterfly clips, so be sure to keep the hair wet enough to stay parted while you cut.

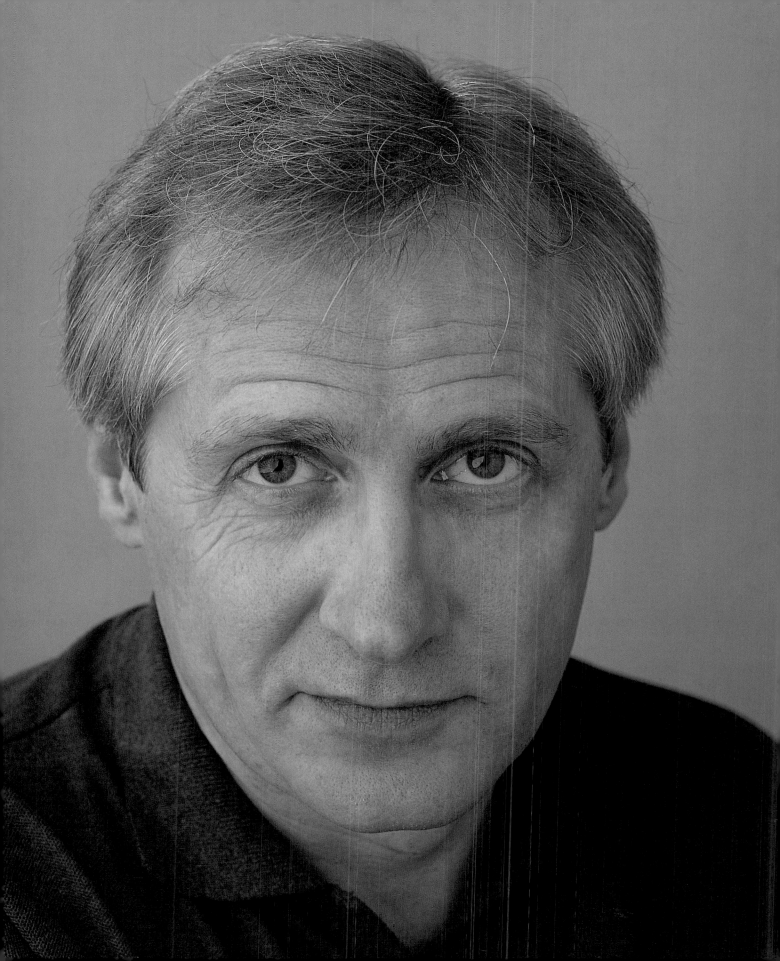

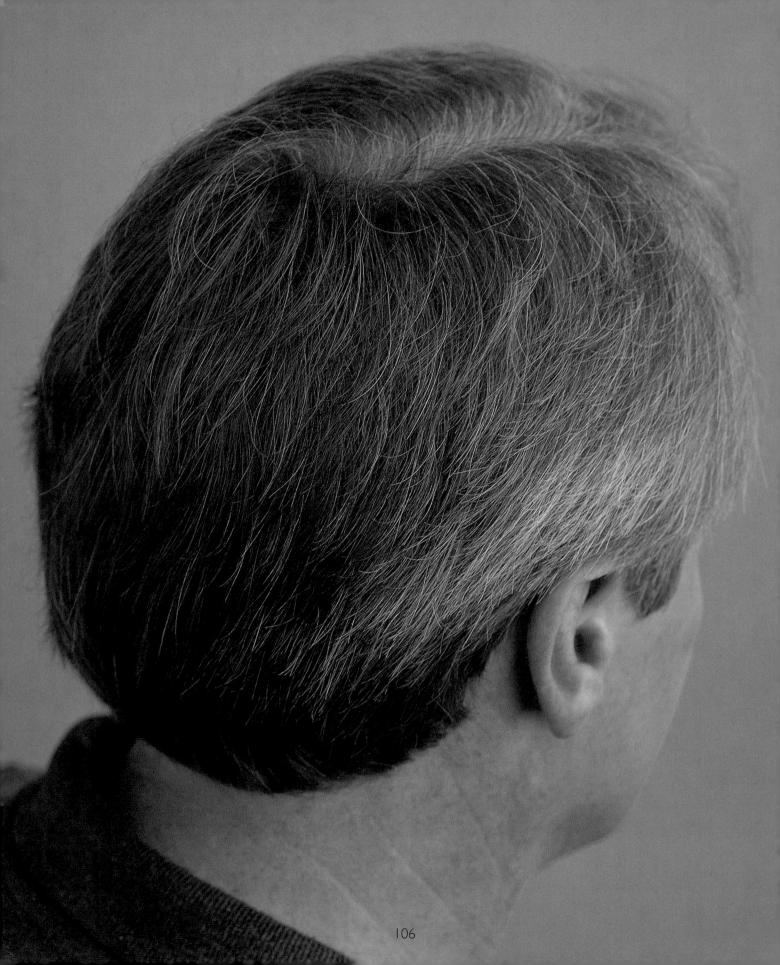

SHORT CUT

Hair Type: Straight hair, fine texture

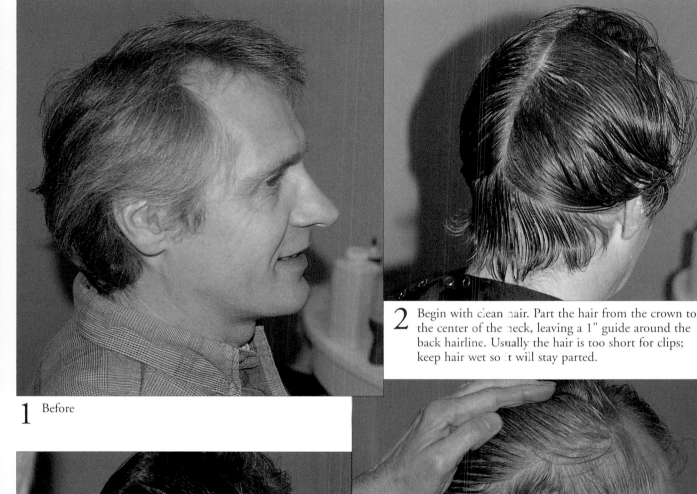

1 Before

2 Begin with clean hair. Part the hair from the crown to the center of the neck, leaving a 1" guide around the back hairline. Usually the hair is too short for clips; keep hair wet so it will stay parted.

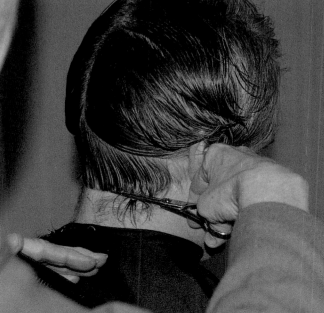

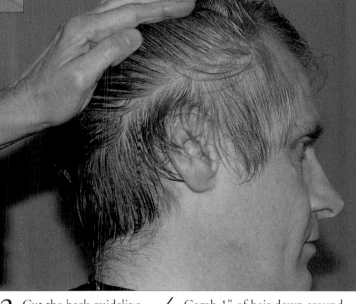

3 Cut the back guideline to the desired length.

continued on page 109

4 Comb 1" of hair down around the ear.

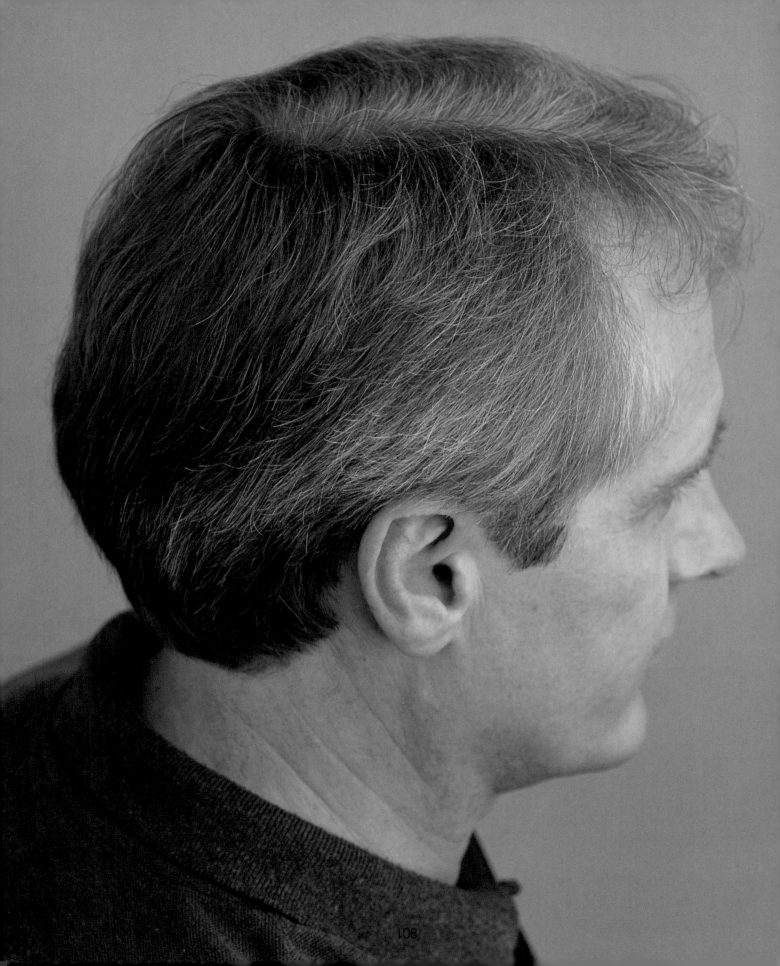

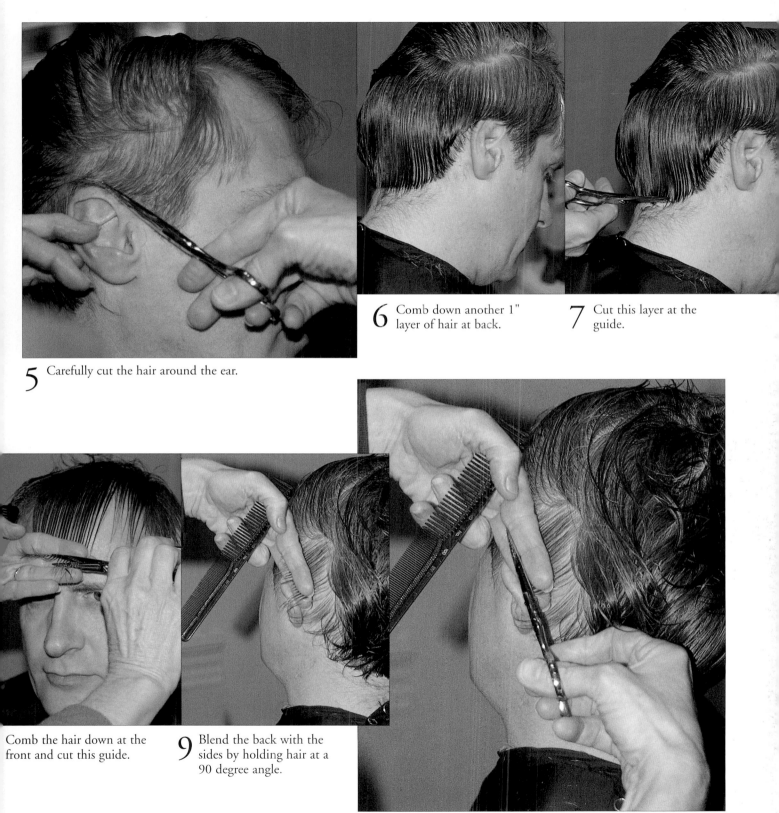

5 Carefully cut the hair around the ear.

6 Comb down another 1" layer of hair at back.

7 Cut this layer at the guide.

Comb the hair down at the front and cut this guide.

9 Blend the back with the sides by holding hair at a 90 degree angle.

10 Cut to guide length.

continued on next page

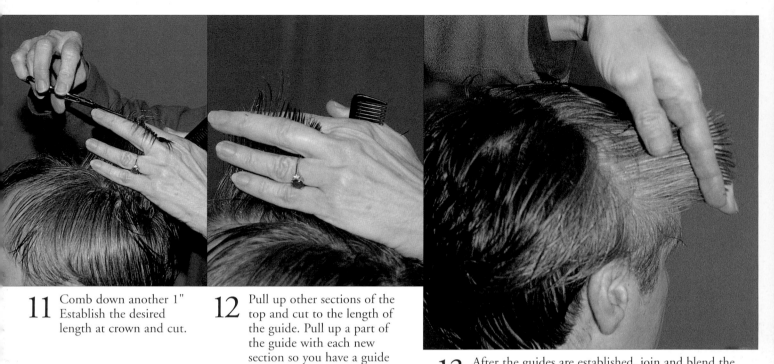

11 Comb down another 1" Establish the desired length at crown and cut.

12 Pull up other sections of the top and cut to the length of the guide. Pull up a part of the guide with each new section so you have a guide to cut to.

13 After the guides are established, join and blend the sections by cutting all of them to the length of the guides.

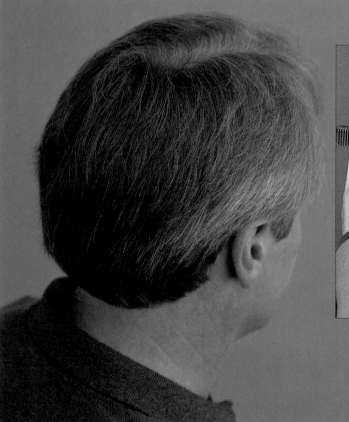

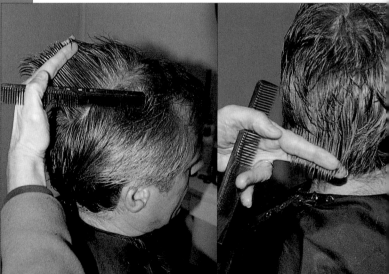

14 Blend the top to the back.

15 Keep blending as you move down, checking the length. When cut is finished the neck can be tidied up with clippers.

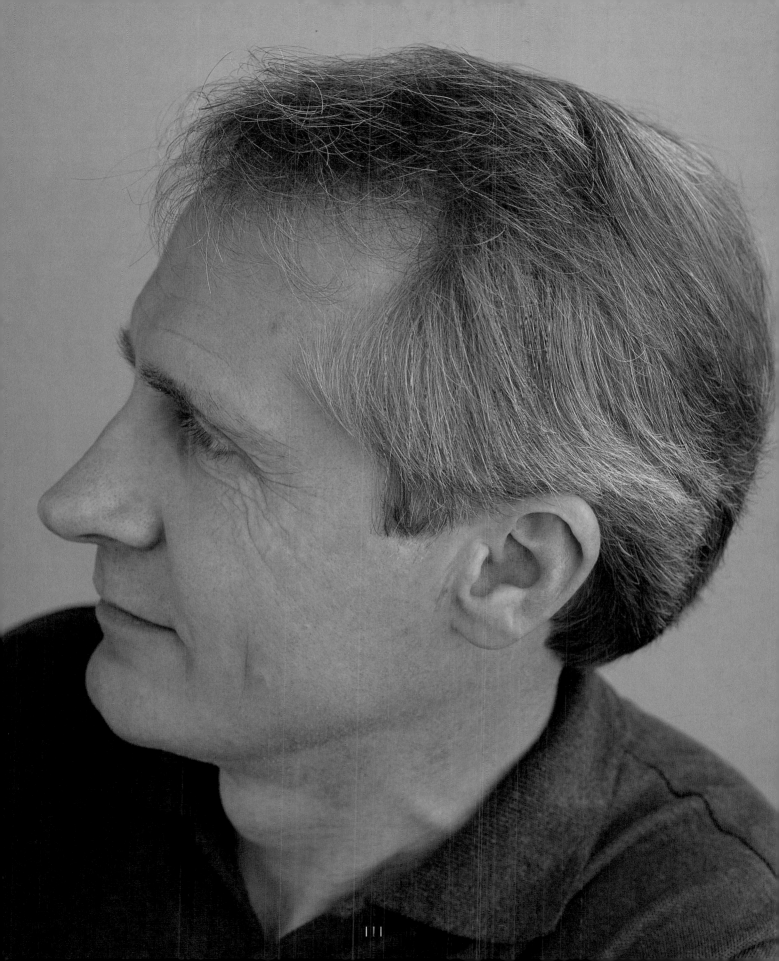

SHORT LAYERED CUT

Hair Type: Thick, wavy

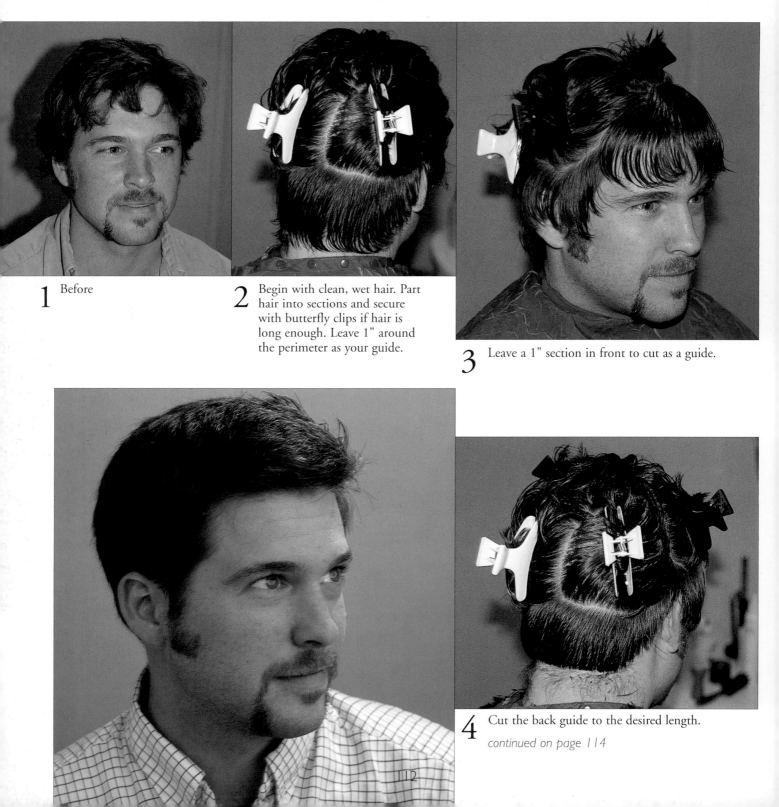

1 Before

2 Begin with clean, wet hair. Part hair into sections and secure with butterfly clips if hair is long enough. Leave 1" around the perimeter as your guide.

3 Leave a 1" section in front to cut as a guide.

4 Cut the back guide to the desired length.

continued on page 114

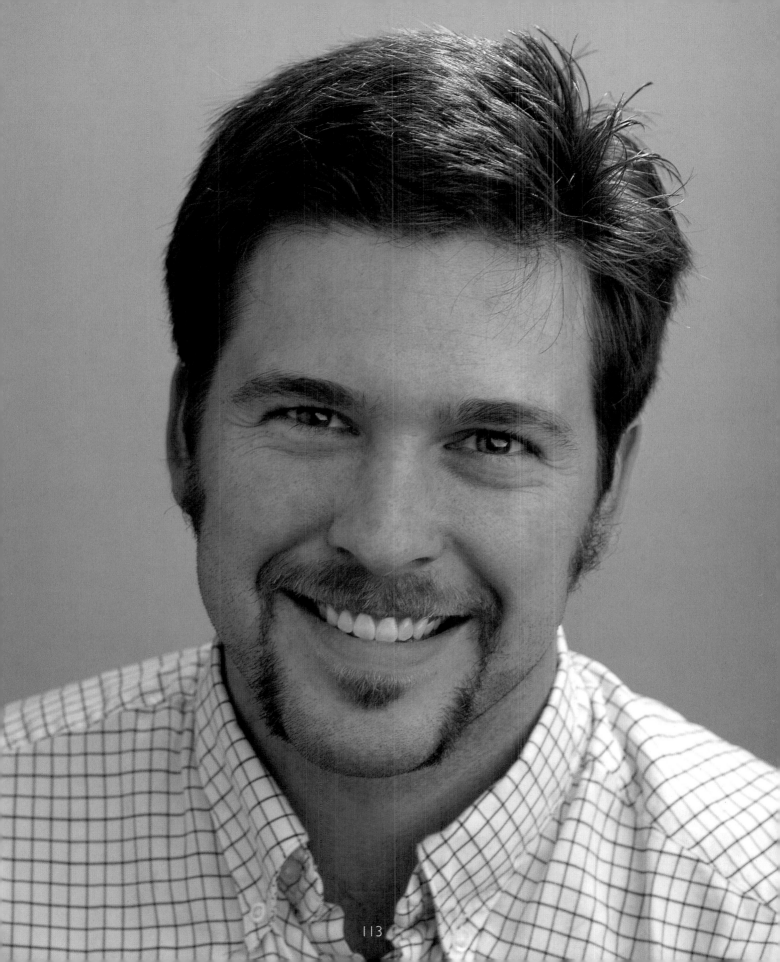

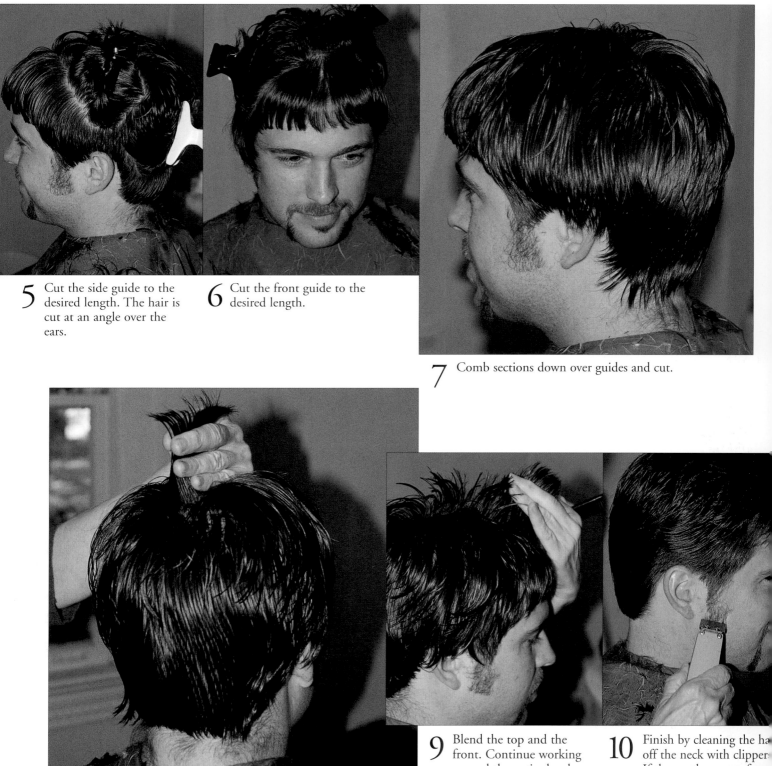

5 Cut the side guide to the desired length. The hair is cut at an angle over the ears.

6 Cut the front guide to the desired length.

7 Comb sections down over guides and cut.

8 Hold hair straight up from the crown and cut to desired length. Continue cutting other top sections. Hold other top sections along with some of the guide straight up and cut to the length of guide.

9 Blend the top and the front. Continue working around the entire head.

10 Finish by cleaning the ha off the neck with clipper If the gentleman prefers sideburns, use clippers to cut these.

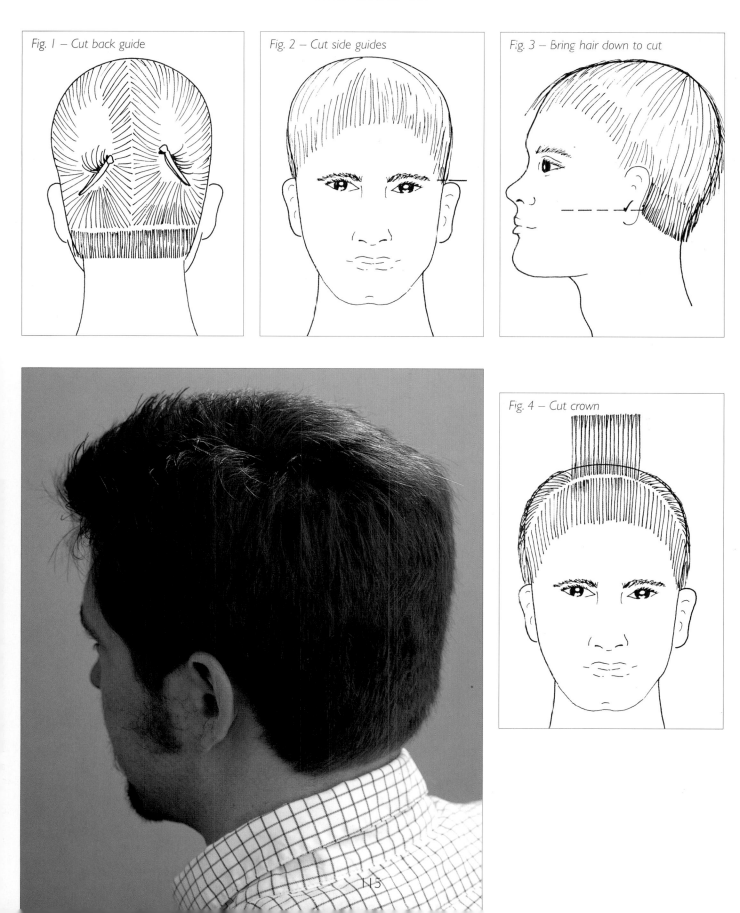

Fig. 1 – Cut back guide

Fig. 2 – Cut side guides

Fig. 3 – Bring hair down to cut

Fig. 4 – Cut crown

MEDIUM LAYERED CUT

Hair Type: Wavy, medium texture

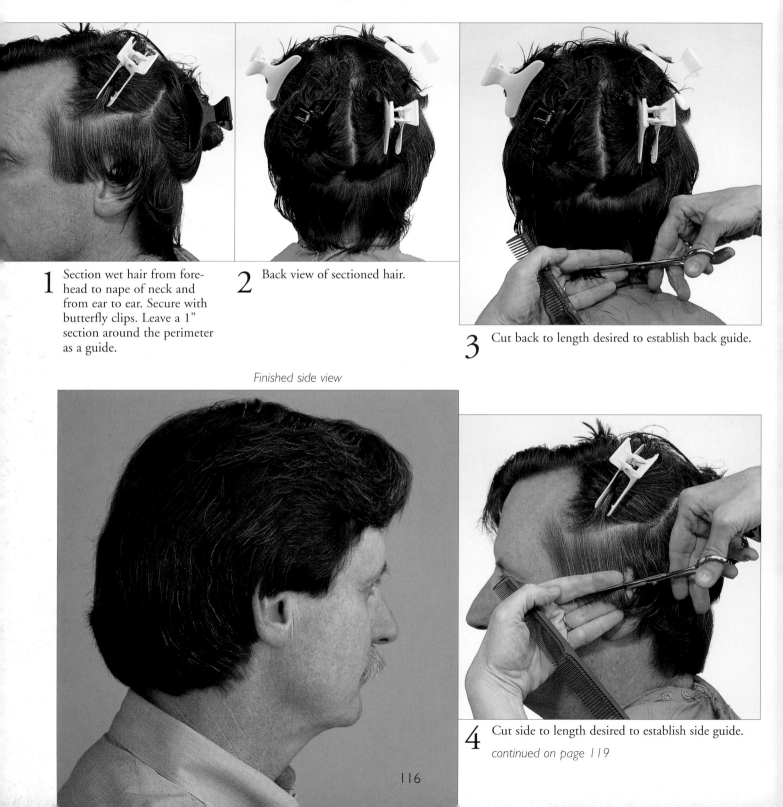

1 Section wet hair from forehead to nape of neck and from ear to ear. Secure with butterfly clips. Leave a 1" section around the perimeter as a guide.

2 Back view of sectioned hair.

3 Cut back to length desired to establish back guide.

Finished side view

4 Cut side to length desired to establish side guide.

continued on page 119

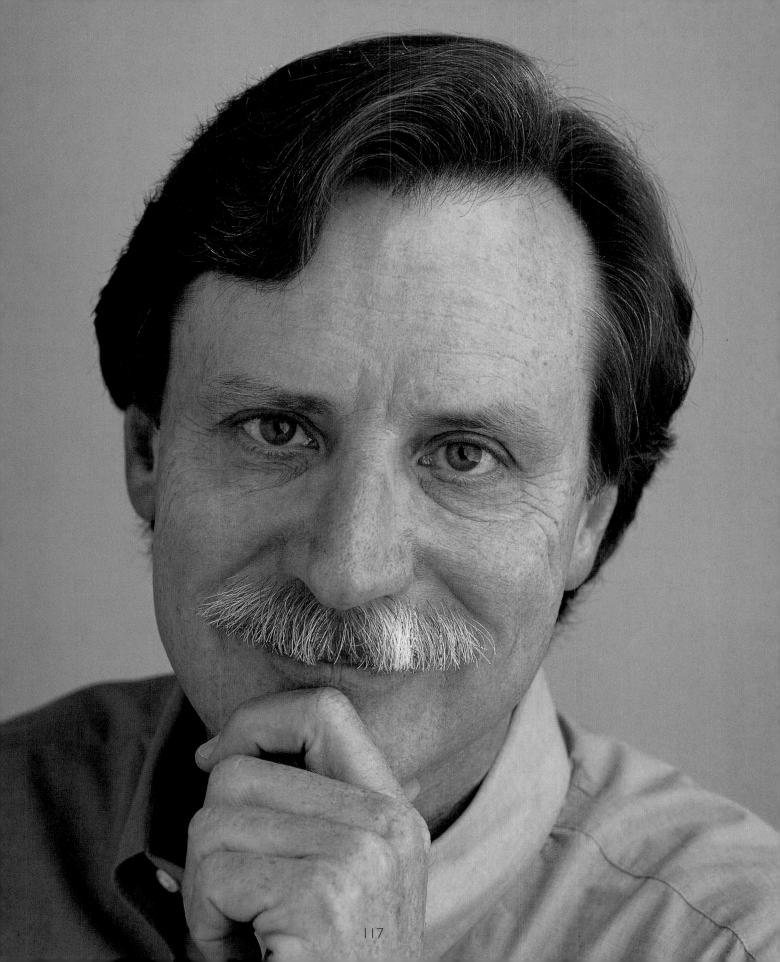

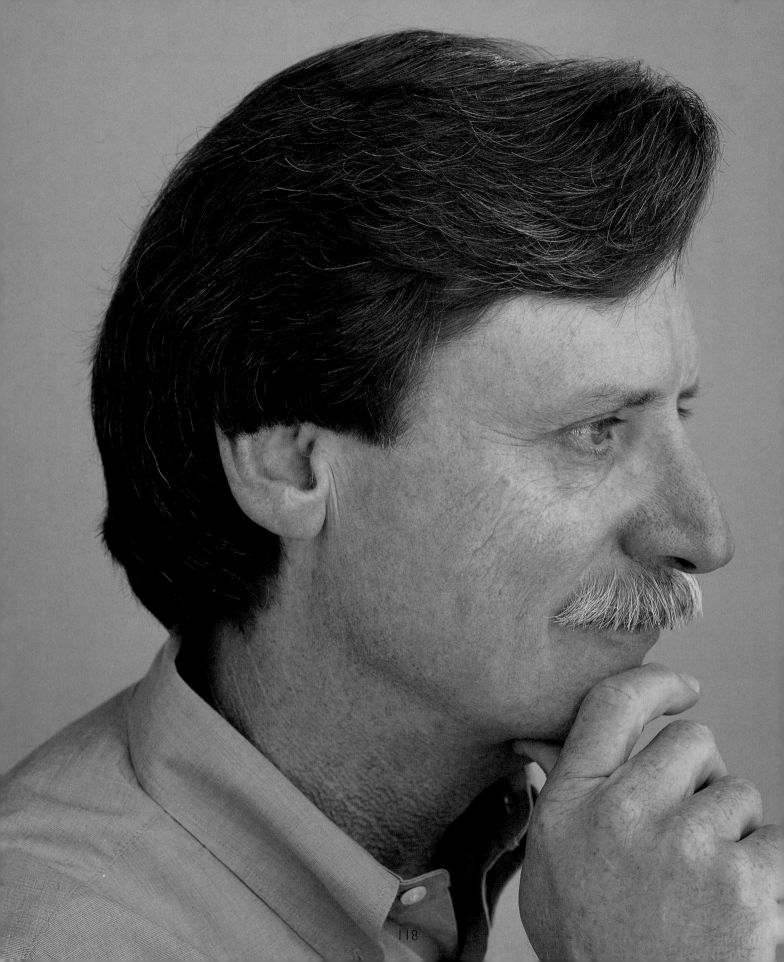

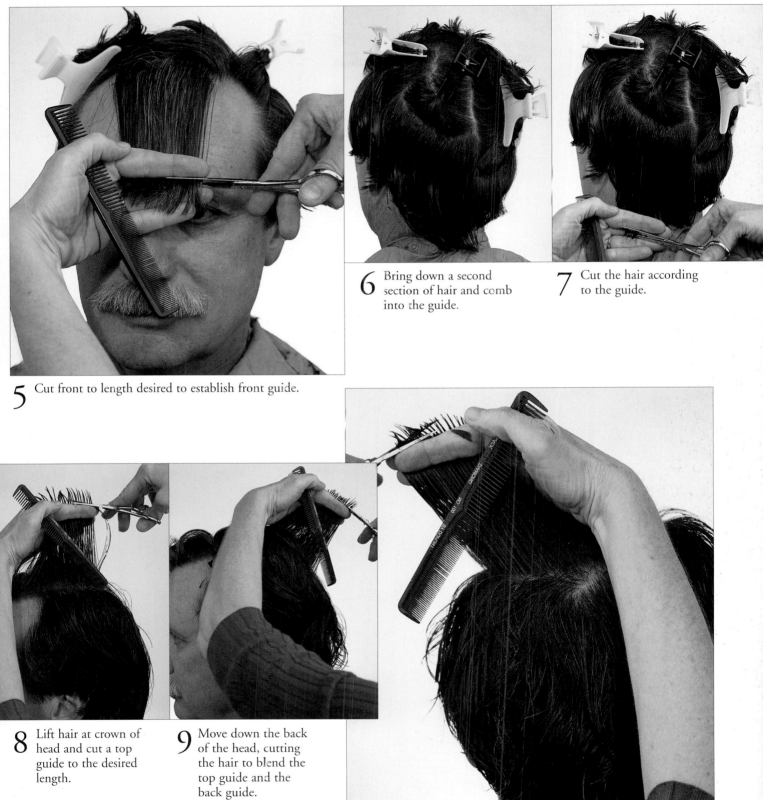

5 Cut front to length desired to establish front guide.

6 Bring down a second section of hair and comb into the guide.

7 Cut the hair according to the guide.

8 Lift hair at crown of head and cut a top guide to the desired length.

9 Move down the back of the head, cutting the hair to blend the top guide and the back guide.

10 Continue to cut, working one section at a time, to blend the top and the back.

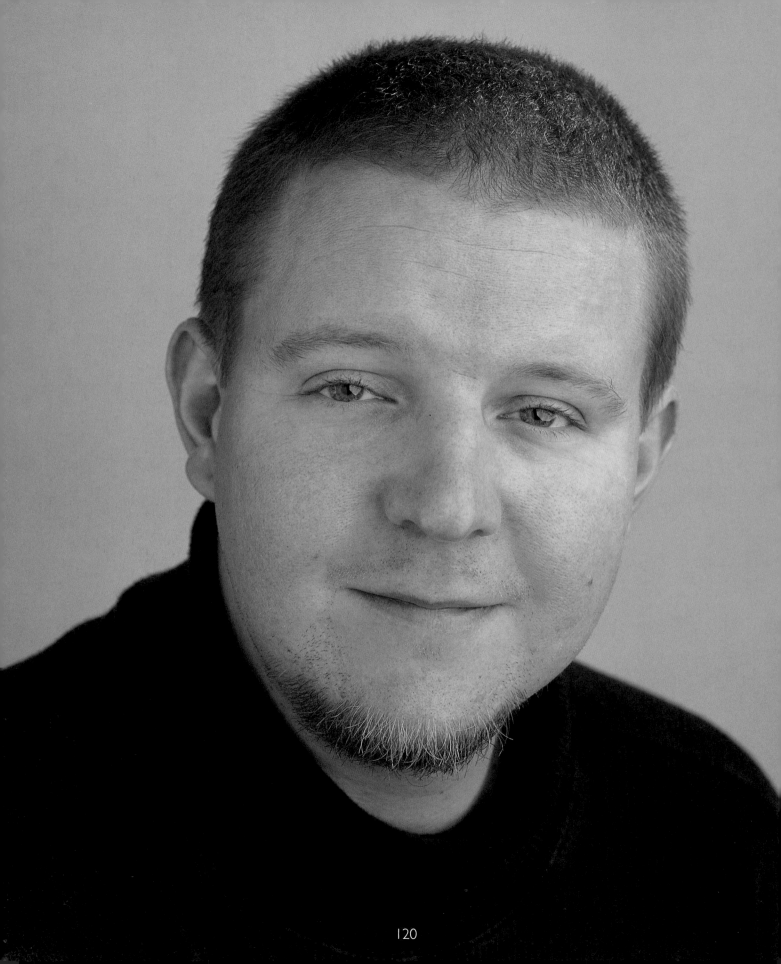

CLIPPER CUT

This haircut is excellent for boys (and many women like it, too). The sides and bottom part of the back are cut with clippers, while the top and the upper part of the back are cut with scissors.

Hair Type: Slightly wavy, medium texture

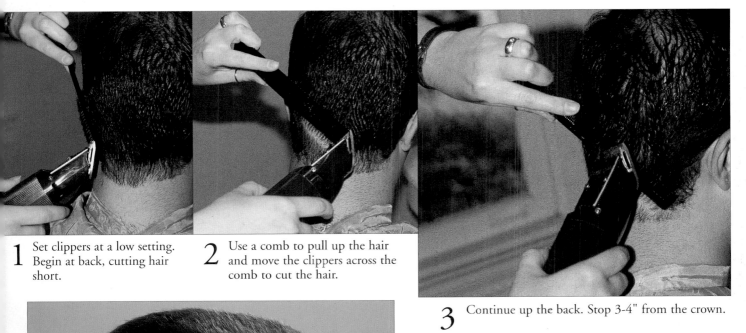

1 Set clippers at a low setting. Begin at back, cutting hair short.

2 Use a comb to pull up the hair and move the clippers across the comb to cut the hair.

3 Continue up the back. Stop 3-4" from the crown.

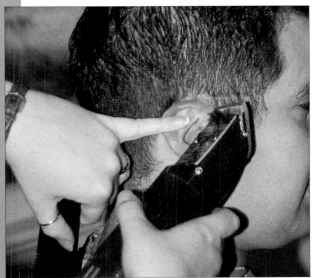

4 Move to the sides, using the clippers to trim the hair above the ears.

continued on next page

Finished side view

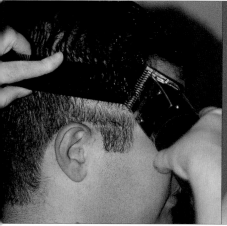

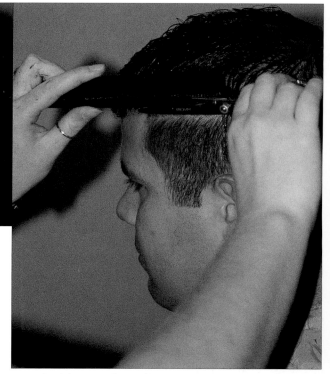

5 Continue clipping up the sides 2-3". Leave the top hair to be cut with scissors. Move around to the back, being sure all the clipped hair is the same length.

6 Cut hair at top back, pulling out hair with your fingers and cutting it to a one-finger length.

7 At sides just above clipper-cut area, use a comb to pull out hair and cut. (A one-finger length is too long at the sides.)

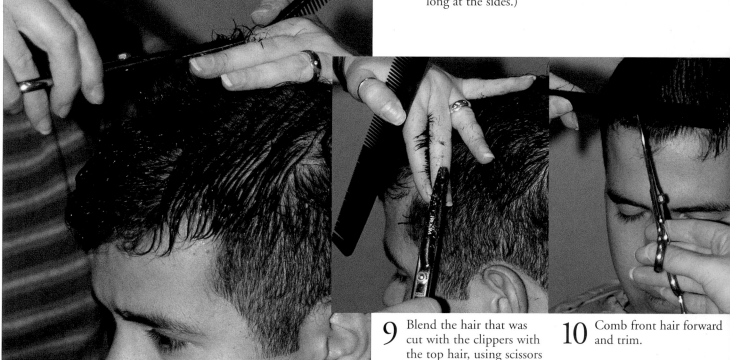

8 Cut the top guide line to the desired length, beginning at the crown. Here, it's cut to a one-finger length. Cut all top hair to this length.

9 Blend the hair that was cut with the clippers with the top hair, using scissors and comb.

10 Comb front hair forward and trim.

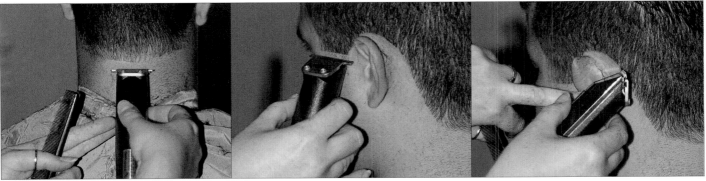

11 Trim across the bottom of the back with clippers.

12 Use clippers to trim sideburns.

13 Hold ears forward and use clippers to tidy up behind the ears.

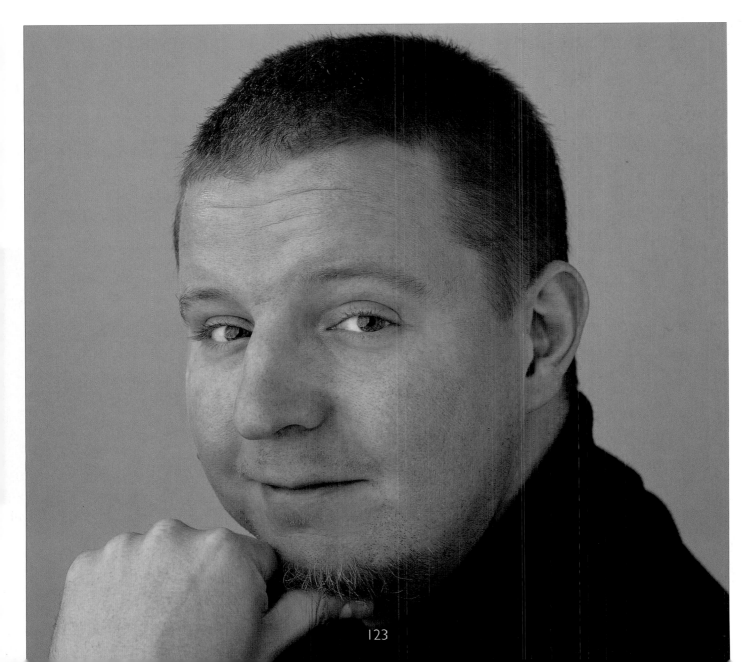

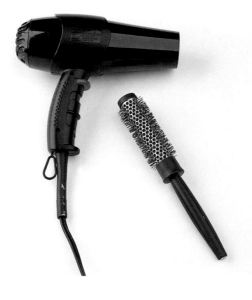

Styling Tips

The cut is the most important part of your style, and certain cuts are more versatile than others. Finishing your style will be easy with the right cut, tools, and products.

Optional styling tools and products are: a blow dryer with a diffuser attachment (an attachment that disperses the air and allows the style to dry undisturbed), a round brush for styling while blow drying, styling gel or mousse, and hair spray.

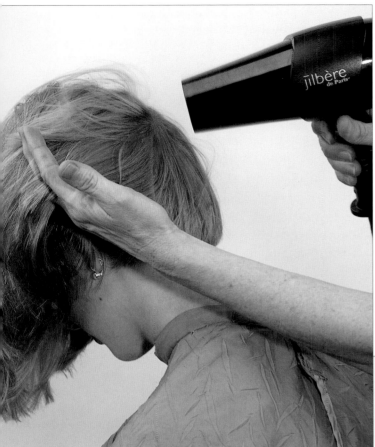

AIR DRYING

Many cuts can be **air dried**, which is desirable because heat damages the hair when used too often and without proper care. When air drying, comb a mousse or gel into the hair and place or mold the hair in the desired style. Allow to dry naturally. When dry fluff up with fingers or comb. A little hair spray will keep the style in place.

BLOW DRYING

Blow drying the hair will give the hair volume and the style you desire can be controlled better. Wet hair thoroughly and then towel dry. Begin blow drying by fluffing the hair with the fingers as you move the air flow about the head. For more volume, turn the head upside down and point air flow at the roots. When the hair is still damp, turn right

Continued on next page

Photo above: Begin by fluffing the hair with the hands as you move blow dryer. dry roots first.

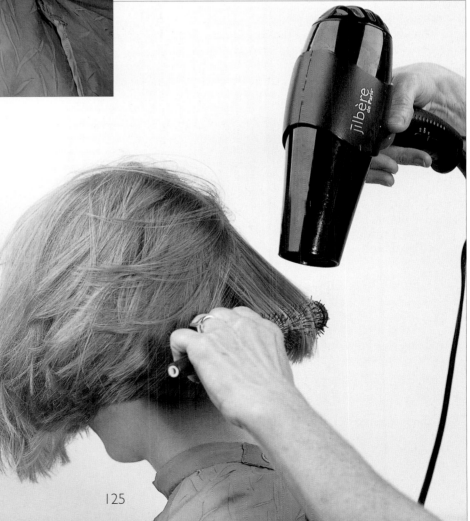

Photo at right: The hair can be styled with the help of a round brush as you use the dryer heat to "set" the style.

125

Blow Drying (cont.)

side up and add mousse or gel. Use a diffuser to continue the drying process, or use a round brush to style.

Blow drying with a brush is a common method for drying hair. Start by applying a styling aid of choice – a mousse or light gel is best. As the styling aid helps the hair glide smoothly around your brush, choose a product that is not sticky or heavy. Using a round brush, take small sections of hair in the brush. Hold the blow dryer in your opposite hand and direct the heat to the brush while turning your wrist. (This takes practice.) Move around the head, turning the hair with the brush to create the desired style and moving the hair in the direction you want it to fall.
• The size of the brush is very important. A smaller brush will give more body and curl, while a larger brush will give a straighter, smoother look.
• Be sure you allow the hair to cool on the brush before removing the brush – this sets the curl and allows the cuticle of the hair to close, causing less damage.

Scrunch drying is another method. This is done with a diffuser. This method usually requires heavier styling aids (mousses, gels, or pomades) and works best on curly or wavy hair. Apply the styling aid and taking the hair in your hand, crumpling it as if it were a piece of paper in your hand as you blow dry.

Hair Protection: There are commercial products for protecting the hair from intense heat. A small amount of oil (such as coconut oil) also can be used.

STYLING TOOLS

✂ Hair Spray

Spraying the hair with a hair spray will set and keep the style. For more volume, spray the hair underneath at roots. Smooth the hair down, brush in place, then spray the surface lightly.

✂ Hair Gel

Here is a recipe for home made hair gel that is a great aid to styling.

✂ Curlers & Curling Irons

Body and curls can be added to fine or straight hair with rollers or curling irons, which are available in numerous sizes. Electric rollers are easy to use and can save time. If you use hot rollers and irons frequently, use a protective product on the hair and condition the hair often. Using the largest rollers or irons will give the hair body. Large rollers will give a smoother, less curled look. If you want tighter curls, use a smaller barrel curling iron or smaller rollers. A heavier styling gel or mousse will help the style last longer.

Flax Seed Hair Gel

Ingredients:
2 tablespoons flax seeds
1 cup distilled water
Optional: A few drops of your favorite essential oil.

Place flax seeds and water in a saucepan. Bring to a boil. Remove from heat and let stand 15 to 20 minutes. Strain. Allow to cool completely. Add essential oil, if desired, to give the gel a nice smell. Store in a glass container.

Contributed by Lisa Van den Boomen

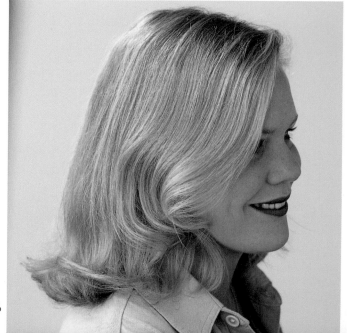

Metric Conversion Chart

Inches to Millimeters and Centimeters				Yards to Meters	
Inches	MM	CM		Yards	Meters
1/8	3	.3		1/8	.11
1/4	6	.6		1/4	.23
3/8	10	1.0		3/8	.34
1/2	13	1.3		1/2	.46
5/8	16	1.6		5/8	.57
3/4	19	1.9		3/4	.69
7/8	22	2.2		7/8	.80
1	25	2.5		1	.91
1-1/4	32	3.2		2	1.83
1-1/2	38	3.8		3	2.74
1-3/4	44	4.4		4	3.66
2	51	5.1		5	4.57
3	76	7.6		6	5.49
4	102	10.2		7	6.40
5	127	12.7		8	7.32
6	152	15.2		9	8.23
7	178	17.8		10	9.14
8	203	20.3			
9	229	22.9			
10	254	25.4			
11	279	27.9			
12	305	30.5			

INDEX